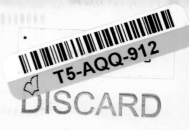

DISCARD

Karlen, Arno.

Napoleon's glands

DATE			

Napoleon's Glands

by cArno Karlen

Napoleon's Glands
and Other Ventures
in Biohistory

by ARNO KARLEN

LITTLE, BROWN AND COMPANY • BOSTON • TORONTO

FIRST EDITION

LIBRARY OF CONGRESS CATALOGING IN PUBLICATION DATA

Karlen, Arno.
  Napoleon's Glands.

  Bibliography: p.
  Includes index.
    1. Diseases and history. 2. Medicine—Miscellanea.
I. Title. II. Title: Biohistory.
R702.K37 1984   900   84-10041
ISBN 0-316-48319-2

BP
Published simultaneously in Canada
by Little, Brown & Company (Canada) Limited
PRINTED IN THE UNITED STATES OF AMERICA

To: Progenitors, Inheritors — and Barbara

Contents

Napoleon's Glands

Introduction

THE ODD ALLURE

IN my early teens, I experienced one of my first thrills of intellectual pleasure while reading a medical biography of Napoleon. The author, an endocrinologist, argued that Bonaparte had conquered and lost empires because of an abnormal thyroid. First the overactive gland drove him to frantic greatness; then the exhausted organ's lethargy cast him into failure and defeat. The doctor took several hundred pages to mesh his medical and historical arguments, showing how the emperor's hormonal problems had become those of the world. The idea seemed marvelously neat, dramatic, and true.

Today I am less convinced, partly on the demerits of the case, partly because I have read an equally exhaustive argument that the key to Napoleon was not his thyroid but a laggard pituitary, and another that the guilty glands were really his allegedly tiny testicles. I have read similar theses that Plotinus's philosophy was the sublime blossom of opium addiction; that El Greco owed his late style, with its flickering slim figures, less to inspiration than to astigmatism; that Dante's genius was announced by the shape of his occiput; that Hitler lost the battle of Stalingrad because of stubborn rage caused by constipation.

Shades of Napoleon's glands! Simplistic, even crankish, as such theories seem, they have an odd allure. It is fascinating to see medicine, biology, history, and other specialized knowledge dovetail, reflecting the complex interweavings of life. There is delight in following intellectual detective work — especially when it seems to hand us a hidden, decisive way to decipher the mysteries of health, behavior, and history. We also have unquenchable, primitive curiosity about our bodies and about famous people. Most important, such theories appeal to a commonsense conviction that the body helps shape personality and behavior.

We have long sought the roots of character and action in the flesh. The search has led through humoral theory, phrenology, and palmistry to somatotyping, behavior genetics, and neuroendocrinology. It seems logical that aches or itches which distract ordinary citizens from business or love affairs may become, in chiefs of state, forces of history. We know that an adrenal tumor can cause psychosis; lead poisoning can induce hallucinations; tuberculosis rings extraordinary changes on mood and personality. Certainly Franklin D. Roosevelt's life was deeply influenced by polio, Edison's by deafness, Dostoevski's by epilepsy. Furthermore, this century has brought vastly increased appreciation of how social and psychological forces influence the body. The social and behavioral sciences, including the new field of psychohistory, have become part of the search to understand human history, human health, and the human future.

There have been fruitful efforts to understand not only individuals but small and large populations. So-called medical history has usually concentrated on telling how pox, plague, and typhus have wiped out armies and civilizations. This is true, and more of value waits discovery, but there are many other questions. Hereditary conditions have afflicted and shaped families, villages, nations, from the hemophilia of the Romanov dynasty to the sickle-cell anemia that gave black Africans protection against more damaging malaria. Diet, climate, and a variety of biological clocks may strongly affect behavior. Changes in nutrition and technology have reshaped the environments of individuals, societies, and the entire biosphere for tens of thousands of years. Viruses can act like floating bits of genetic material, and the recent explosion of knowledge about them suggests startling ideas about our species' origins and future.

There have been few attempts to integrate our growing information from the medical, biological, and behavioral sciences and use it in interpreting the human past. This effort I call biohistory. It goes beyond collecting curiosa about the ills of the famous and anecdotes about plagues of the past. Biohistory draws on medical history, psychohistory, archaeology, biology, ecology, psychiatry — every view of the human social animal — to study the past and its relation to our present and future. It examines individuals, families, populations, and our species as it evolves along with its ecosystem. To give just a few examples, it can:

— by studying fracture patterns and growth-lines in bones from prehistoric sites, deduce the extent of a vanished people's aggression, their nutrition and health, the sexual division of labor, and sometimes technology, religion, and more.

— combine the history of science, the history of art, and modern medical knowledge to examine the idea that creative genius contains a kernel of pathology.

— by blood-typing ancient mummies and contemporary people, learn how cultures without written history have evolved physically and culturally, and how they have migrated and mixed with other peoples over millennia.

— anticipate how chemical contraceptives may change men's and women's emotional interaction, sexual selection, and thus the human evolutionary future.

The scope of biohistory is vast. The first few chapters of this book use studies in individual biography to explore the biohistorian's tools and methods. Later chapters go beyond individuals, applying these tools to communities and large populations. The final sections broaden the view to the human species and its environment. Each chapter is a case study showing some of the subjects, techniques, and possibilities of this interdisciplinary venture. The bibliography, though not exhaustive or complete by formal scholarly standards, gives the reader a springboard to further pursue biohistory.

All of this leaps far beyond my own first case in biohistory, the question of whether Napoleon's glands or other organs are truly a significant part of history. This is a good introduction to the puzzle-solving nature of biohistory, its uses, abuses, and fascination.

1

Napoleon's Glands

THE GREAT MAN'S ITCH

Napoleon's life and health raise the simplest, most common question people have asked of biohistory — whether a great man's itch really does force millions to scratch. The metaphor is not arbitrary. Many of us first heard of Napoleon's ills in the joking or serious story that he kept one hand inside his coat to scratch himself or to hold an aching stomach. When I first heard this lore, in grade school, the alleged reasons were lice or "executive ulcer." In fact, Napoleon did suffer dreadful itching and gastric upsets, and they affected more than his poses.

Napoleon claimed that he caught scabies, a highly contagious skin disease commonly called "the itch," during the siege of Toulon in 1793. This may be true, but he also suffered severe neurodermatitis, or nervous itching, on and off throughout his life. This often results from compulsive scratching when under stress. Napoleon once said, "I live only by my skin." He was known to scratch pimples on his face till they bled so badly that soldiers wondered whether he had been wounded. Under tension he sometimes clawed at an old leg wound; at least once he did so till blood gushed forth — "to open a vent" (presumably

for noxious humors), said Napoleon. The long baths he
took may have been partly to relieve his dermal distress.
He may have used other stress relievers; Lewis Way, in
his book *Adler's Place in Psychology,* says Napoleon mas-
turbated before battle to release some of his enormous
tension.

Bonaparte's crackling energy and his life of constant
crisis provoked other symptoms. He suffered rages, weep-
ing, twitches, migrainelike headaches, blackouts, fits. There
was also a more private and humiliating symptom, which
Dr. William Ober says explains the "enigma of Waterloo," Napoleon's strange failure to pursue his initial advantage in that battle. One must hear out the argument
before scoffing at the post-postmortem diagnosis in Ober's
essay "Seats of the Mighty" — that Napoleon suffered
agonizing hemorrhoids that helped dethrone him at Waterloo.

Napoleon's attacks of hemorrhoids, like his nervous itch,
often came before and during battles, the times when
soldiers receive the traditional warning, "Keep a tight
asshole!" Trying to control stress and strong emotion does
tend to tighten the anus; prolonged tension and straining
at stool can cause throbbing varicose veins, fistulas, and
other damage to the sensitive ano-rectal tissues. Irregular
eating, constipation, and infrequent bathing — all conditions of combat and crisis — help cause or aggravate
such ills. The one American in four who has experienced
a hemorrhoid or fistula knows it is funny only to the other
three. Sitting can be agony, walking a torment; finally any
posture, even lying down, is misery. Burning pain becomes one's shadow, producing rage, outrage, and exhaustion. One of the few reliefs from hemorrhoids is long
hot baths, perhaps a better reason than scabies for Napoleon's devotion to the tub.

Napoleon had severe attacks of hemorrhoids from his late twenties until the end of his military career; there was a dreadful bout during the Russian campaign and a possibly fateful one in 1815. In that last year he escaped from Elba and traveled across the Alps to reach Paris; during this journey he suffered a mild attack. It subsided in Paris while he planned for battle, but it resumed in full force around June 13, on the road to Waterloo. Riding horseback with piles is a fate to be wished on one's worst enemy. That is just what Napoleon did all day before the battle.

The French won an advantage at Ligny on June 17. Normally Napoleon would have capitalized on it speedily. Instead, he lay awake much of the night in pain and finally arose, exhausted and sluggish, at eight o'clock. To his generals' frustration, he issued no orders for several hours; meanwhile the opposing Allies repositioned themselves, and the French advantage was gone. Throughout the day, Napoleon seemed foggy, erratic, indecisive; some of his actions still puzzle historians. At one point he dismounted and stood clutching a fence post, his face white with pain, and for an hour he straddled a chair by the road to Brussels. Wellington later said Waterloo was one of the narrowest victories he had seen. Napoleon's fatigue, pain, and limited mobility could have made the difference. Dr. Ober says:

"One cannot rewrite history, and there is no guarantee that Napoleon would have defeated Wellington and Blücher if he had not suffered from acutely thrombosed hemorrhoids, but in the long run one cannot consider it safe for an empire to rest on so sensitive and fragile a bottom." He goes on to quote the Bible on how the Lord unseats the mighty: "*Deposuit potentes de sede* has been said of the Almighty, but hemorrhoids can play their part."

Readers who think this is a tunnel vision of history

should consider the case of Louis XIV of France. He
suffered many ills, but the most painful was piles. These
began when he was in his early thirties and after some
fifteen years were complicated by a wretched anal fistula.
When in pain, Louis went into explosive rages, and the
public weal may have suffered proportionately. The royal
malady was finally cured by surgery, after which Louis
enjoyed thirty years of good health and relatively good
temper. (There were then, as always, people ready to
follow a leader anywhere; some perfectly healthy courtiers
ran for fistulotomies.) We prefer to think the mind rules
human fate, but the great historian Michelet considered
Louis's recovery from chronic rectal pain the turning point
of his reign. I, for one, would not care to be ruled by a
man with a chronic toothache, let alone a rectal fistula.

Those who still doubt that Napoleon's end was his nemesis should ponder another privy ill: The cries of pain
heard through Napoleon's bathroom door were sometimes
caused by dysuria, or urinary pain. Only a handful of
people knew this while Napoleon lived, and he made them
swear to keep it secret, which they did for fifty years. Sir
Walter Scott's nine-volume biography of Napoleon, published in 1827, doesn't mention this malady. But Hugo's
Les Misérables, a few decades later, said that on the second day of Waterloo Napoleon suffered "local trouble"
and rode through the day with "ghastly bladder pain."

Sharp dysuria struck Bonaparte as early as 1800, at the
battle of Marengo, and recurred all his life, often at critical
moments. During the Russian campaign, at Borodino, his
pain was dreadful as he forced out urine in drops heavy
with sediment. During six years of captivity on St. Helena,
he was often seen leaning his head against a tree, trying
in vain to urinate. The pain became so sharp that he rarely
slept more than a few hours at a time and often quit

meetings abruptly. He once told his last physician, Francesco Antommarchi, "This is my weak spot, and it will ultimately cause my death."

There were two reasons for Napoleon's secrecy about his bladder trouble. One was his difficulty producing heirs during his marriage to Josephine; for many years he was sensitive about anything that might cast doubt on his potency and genital health. The other was the rumor that he returned to Josephine from a long military campaign with venereal disease. His doctors insisted to gossipers that it wasn't true, but to little effect. Talk of an "amatory complaint" rose again when the Allied Commissioners were taking him to exile on Elba. The accuser, the Prussian Count Truchsess von Waldburg, may have inferred venereal infection from Napoleon's urinary problem. There is no convincing evidence that Napoleon ever had gonorrhea or syphilis, but the idea recurred sporadically before and after his death. The postmortem showed gravel and small stones in a diseased bladder, cause enough for his urinary pain.

Dermatitis, piles, and urinary pain weren't Napoleon's only barometers of stress. His physician in the field from 1796 till 1814, Dr. Yvan, wrote that "The emperor's constitution was highly nervous. He was very susceptible to emotional influences, and the spasm was ordinarily divided between the stomach and the bladder." His stomach, like his bladder, probably cost him some battles. In 1813, on the verge of routing the Allies at Dresden, he was prostrated by stomach pain and vomiting, and he had to give command to subordinates, who botched his good start. Two months later, a similar attack flattened him at the battle of Leipzig. He also sometimes had an exhausting cough, perhaps psychosomatic, perhaps the result of mild tubercular or other lung infection. Finally, there was some other internal pain. Napoleon's secretary, Fauvelet de Bourrienne, recorded that early in 1802 the emperor began to suffer such pain in the right side that it made him irritable and probably affected some of his decisions (this conclusion is de Bourrienne's). Often Napoleon unbuttoned his waistcoat, leaned on the right arm of his chair, and exclaimed how severe the pain was. He started keeping his hand inside his coat to hold the aching spot.

Some of Napoleon's abdominal pain seems to have been in the region of his liver, some in the stomach. When he was very sick on St. Helena, and his stomach trouble terribly acute, Napoleon told his doctor that his father had died in his late thirties of stomach cancer, and he worried about the disease running in his family. Therefore he asked that an autopsy be done and the results sent to his son. The autopsy did lead to the conclusion that stomach cancer was the immediate cause of his death, but from that day till the present, dissenters have suspected other ills, and some have suggested direct or indirect murder.

The case remains alive because Napoleon's life, health, and death were always fraught with political implications; in his late years these matters were potential propaganda dynamite. Imagine that Hitler survived World War II and was banished to a small Mediterranean island, watched over by British officials and doctors. Enemies, followers, victims of Nazis, and crypto-Nazis all over the world would see danger or reassurance in his every sniffle or healthy day. The world would hang on the slightest rumor, and nations everywhere would see threat or promise in his treatment or mistreatment, his life and death. Probably no account would satisfy everyone. That was just the case with Napoleon.

Arguments began about St. Helena itself as soon as it was chosen for Napoleon's banishment. Many Frenchmen feared Napoleon had been sent to a semitropical pesthole to perish conveniently of real or alleged diseases. Pope Pius VII, once arrested and humiliated by Napoleon, asked that he be released, because he thought "the craggy island of St. Helena mortally injurious to health . . . the poor exile is dying by inches." Sir Walter Scott later called the place a "devil's island," its governor, Sir Hudson Lowe, a "hired assassin."

Predictably, the British tended to exaggerate the island's resemblance to a luxury spa. Actually, the climate was humid but temperate, neither the best nor worst imaginable. Some diseases were common there, as in much of the Mediterranean then, and Napoleon's quarters were uncomfortable and unhygienic. Probably most important to the British, who had seen Napoleon return once from island exile, it was small, out-of-the-way, little visited, a perfect prison without bars for the world's most important captive. In all, Napoleon was treated ungenerously, and the British probably hoped he would finish his days on St. Helena before long; but they probably were not so maladroit as to mistreat him openly.

But in 1816, Napoleon's second year on the island, he developed swollen legs and a dull pain in the right side. Dr. Barry O'Meara of the Royal Navy diagnosed hepatitis and administered purgatives and other futile medications. O'Meara's diagnosis and his growing sympathy with Napoleon set him in conflict with governor Lowe, who in 1818 had him arrested and recalled to England. There O'Meara hinted that Lowe had been ordered to speed up Napoleon's death. O'Meara was dismissed from the navy. Historians usually discredit him as a destructive gossip and perhaps a man of divided political loyalties; still, his worst crime in British eyes was diagnosing hepatitis, giving ammunition to those who claimed Napoleon was being maltreated. O'Meara's offense was soon repeated. Napoleon, whose health had continued to be irregular, had a fainting fit in January 1819. A British navy doctor named John Stokoe was called in and diagnosed hepatitis. Infuriated, Lowe charged him with medical and political blunders; Stokoe was forced to resign from the service. Probably more to Lowe's liking was a visitor from the British Foreign Office who declared Napoleon's illness not hepatic but "diplomatic."

In October 1820, after an interval of relatively good health, Napoleon collapsed after one of his hot baths. He suffered violent vomiting and became increasingly sick and weak. In March of the following year, the British Dr. Arnott joined the Corsican Dr. Antommarchi on the case. He suspected not the liver but the stomach. A few weeks later, Napoleon vomited black fluid, a sign of bleeding in the stomach. Antommarchi made the fantastic decision to administer a harsh emetic; it made Napoleon roll on the floor in agony, but that didn't prevent further dosings. In early April, Napoleon complained of razor-sharp pains in his stomach. Arnott, like Antommarchi, prescribed more purgatives. Today their judgment seems appalling; in fact, purging a patient in Napoleon's condition seems malicious. But in that day, doctors commonly subjected weak or even dying patients to purging, bleeding, and blistering.

Reports on Napoleon's health continued to be shaped by political pressure and medical muddle. In early April, Arnott still claimed the prisoner had only dyspepsia, and his ills were chiefly mental. While Arnott wrote of hypochondria, Napoleon became feverish and feeble, suspected terminal stomach cancer, and wrote a new will. On April 25, he began vomiting what looked like coffee grounds — digested blood, which signals a bleeding ulcer, cancer, or other critical gastrointestinal condition. On May

5, after a week of lapses into unconsciousness and delirium, Napoleon died.

Napoleon had requested an autopsy, and the world expected one.* The emperor's staff and more than a dozen observers, most of them British medical officers, crowded into a billiard room to watch Antommarchi do a job that was not thorough even by the standards of his day. The stomach had a hole "large enough to admit a little finger," but the organ adhered to the liver so that the opening was blocked. Only Napoleon's face and calves were starting to show the ghastly emaciation common in stomach cancer; the bleeding, perforation, and probably peritonitis (perhaps all speeded by purgatives) seem to have spared Napoleon a lingering death. The commonest opinion today remains that Napoleon died of a cancerous, perforated stomach.

The British government and Sir Hudson Lowe must have been happy to say that Napoleon had died of the same disease as his father and several other relatives. But from then till today, a significant minority of doctors and historians have made other claims, ranging from various diseases to malign neglect to outright homicide. Their cases range from earnestly scholarly to patently political.

The most popular second diagnosis involves the alleged hepatitis that ended the careers of two Royal Navy physicians. At the autopsy, Antommarchi examined and cut into Napoleon's liver and declared it congested, enlarged, but without abscess or cancerous growth. Dr. Shortt, one of the observing English doctors, contended that the liver

---

*It is Arnott's testimony that Napoleon feared cancer, Antommarchi's that he asked for an autopsy, and some writers have doubted them both. In fact, there are few fully reliable witnesses to Napoleon's last years. On balance, I think, Antommarchi and especially Arnott can probably be believed on these points.

was "very large, distended with blood . . . and affected by chronic hepatitis." Dr. Arnott and three other British doctors disagreed. Shortt's opinion was struck from the official postmortem report by governor Lowe, and the organ was officially proclaimed "perhaps a little larger than natural."

Further argument arose later, when Antommarchi said in his memoirs that the liver had indeed been affected by chronic hepatitis, and that Napoleon actually died of a chronic gastroenteritis (probably amoebic dysentery) that was common on St. Helena. The question today is whether Antommarchi lied in the autopsy report, attempting to defend St. Helena and the British, or whether he lied later to justify having overlooked the cancer symptoms. O'Meara and others had written that St. Helena was notorious for gastroenteritis; Sir Walter Scott, visiting St. Helena not many years after Napoleon's death, found in the hospital there not one record of it. Some French historians have argued that such records are easily altered.

There are writers who still argue that St. Helena was indeed a sink of hepatitis, dysentery, and medical neglect. The French physician R. Brice and the American Ralph Korngold have written in recent decades that Napoleon died of a liver abscess caused by amoebic hepatitis. A French doctor named Abbatucci fires with two barrels: "Napoleon died from the effects of an abscess of the liver complicated by amoebic dysentery. . . ." Some such writers seem bent at all times on making Napoleon a victim, even a martyr, and one wonders how a fatal liver abscess escaped even unwilling eyes at the autopsy. But the real issue is whether one wants to blame British venom for exposing Napoleon to amoebae that weakened and perhaps killed him.

Some accusations have been stronger, including one by

Bonaparte himself. In a will written a few weeks before his death, he said, "I die prematurely, murdered by the English oligarchy and its hired assassin. The people of England will not fail to avenge me." Like much of the will, this seems a calculated stroke of Napoleon's usual political dramatizing; the will also proclaimed allegiance to a church he privately denied and to a wife who had just become another man's mistress. However, a direct charge of poisoning was finally made in 1962, because of evidence provided by Napoleon himself.

In his will, the dying emperor ordered that his head be shaved and locks of his hair given to some of his retinue. The hair was preserved by two of his valets, and almost a century and a half later, a Swedish dentist with an interest in toxicology named Sten Forshufvud had it subjected to laboratory tests and discovered a high level of arsenic. He pointed out that arsenic can be given in small, unnoticed doses until enough accumulates in the body to be fatal. The internal organs don't last long after death, but the hair and fingernails do, and they retain a predictable portion of the arsenic a person consumed. There the poison can be detected decades or even centuries later. Forshufvud maintained that Napoleon died of chronic arsenic poisoning, deliberate or accidental. He allowed for inadvertance because arsenic was widely used in medicines in Napoleon's day. The arsenic theory drew international attention when it appeared, but it convinced few.

Almost two decades later, Forshufvud's theory again seized wide attention; he had pursued his theory, and two authors wrote a popular book detailing his work. He had had cooperation from other scientists in cutting hairs from Napoleon's head into sections, to determine when in time the arsenic had been absorbed. His final conclusion was that Napoleon had been slowly, systematically poisoned by one of his retinue, acting not on behalf of the English but of the royalist cause in France. As evidence he presented what he considered a conspiratorial effort to hinder his research by French scholars.

When the book *The Murder of Napoleon* appeared with these details in 1982, some reviewers spoke of a masterpiece of forensic medicine finally solving a crime a century and a half old. There were scientists who responded far less favorably. Three researchers studied Napoleon's hair and found only a slight increase in arsenic, but a great increase in antimony, a metal commonly used in medicines in Napoleon's day; it can give false readings of arsenic in laboratory tests. One of the researchers, Dr. Peter Lewin of Toronto, concluded that the poisoning-conspiracy theory should be buried, the old autopsy finding be accepted. A British chemist, David Jones of the University of Newcastle upon Tyne, examined a sample of the wallpaper from the room in which Napoleon died and found that it contained a high, if nonlethal, level of arsenic. Environmental contamination of a body by arsenic, before or after death, has always been one of the problems in postmortem diagnoses of poisoning. So a strong case remains that the level of arsenic in Napoleon's hair was high but not lethal or proof of poisoning.

The arguments for death by hepatitis, dysentery, poisoning, and medical maltreatment all seem to me to have more demerits than merits. However, another theory, ingenious and intellectually appealing, has received some favorable attention since it appeared a decade ago, for it neatly embraces many of Napoleon's ills. Dr. Wardner D. Ayer, in an article in the *N.Y. State Journal of Medicine,* accepted stomach cancer as the cause of death but proposed another clinical villain to explain the hepatitis, dysuria, hemorrhoids, and much more. The disease, schistosomiasis, has been found in the autopsies of mummified ancient pharaohs and perhaps infected Napoleon during his Egyptian campaign.

This parasitic scourge shortens the lives of several hundred million people in tropical and subtropical zones — recently up to 90 percent of black Rhodesians and a quarter of the natives of Puerto Rico and some other Caribbean islands. The cause is the schistosome, a microscopic creature that finds an intermediate host in snails inhabiting stagnant ponds and irrigation ditches. The larvae, or wrigglers, pierce the skin of people working or bathing in the water, enter the bloodstream, and invade the liver, lungs, intestines, and especially the rectum and urinary tract. There they lay tiny spiked eggs, and new parasites appear, generation after generation, causing a great variety of symptoms, weakness, and vulnerability to other disorders. This disease was described in Egyptian papyri more than three thousand years ago, and in an early landmark of biohistory, Marc Armand Ruffer announced in 1910 that he had autopsied six mummies of the Twentieth Dynasty, and in two of them found calcified schistosome eggs. The source of the disease was not recognized until 1851, by Dr. Theodor Bilharz of Berlin. It is called bilharzia after him or schistosomiasis after its cause; British soldiers in Africa dubbed it "Bill Harris," and Napoleon's troops cursed it as "Egyptian hematuria."

Napoleon spent a year and four months in Egypt in 1798–1799. Already in the habit of taking long baths, he may have done so often in infected water. He eventually showed many of the usual symptoms — scalding urinary pain, an enlarged liver, pain in the right side, hemorrhoids, skin rashes, swollen ankles, a dry cough, and gravel in the bladder. All except hemorrhoids began after his return from Egypt. In fact, he had all the major symptoms except, to our knowledge, urinary bleeding. The occasional cough and the so-called tubercles that showed on Napoleon's upper left lung at autopsy may also have resulted from bilharzia. The cough doesn't seem to have brought suggestions of tuberculosis during Napoleon's life, and Dr. Ayer points out that the schistosome's hard, spiked eggs can lodge in the lungs and cause what resemble tubercular nodules. It would take modern microscopic study to know if this was the case, but bilharzia does neatly fit Napoleon's great array of symptoms over two decades.

One would gladly let Napoleon off the diagnostic table at this point, laden with theories of poisoning, piles, and parasites, but another medical question remains, more important than the cause of his death. That is the dramatic change in appearance, personality, and vitality that began during his late thirties. Napoleon affected the world as much as any other man, and his changing health and character affected his leadership. That raises the matter with which we began — Napoleon's glands.

Young Napoleon was slim, hawklike, taut in body and intelligence. Like many men who win great power, he had vast energy that allowed him to work harder and longer than most, with intense concentration and command of numberless details. Sometimes he slept only a few hours a night and took very brief naps through the day. He not only led his troops as a field general but showed superabundant vitality in his intellect and emotions — as a daring tactician, a master of logistics, a politician, a legislator, a manipulator of individuals and crowds. Napoleon had nerve, dash, and a brilliant theatrical sense, from rages that he turned on and off as needed to a charm that won not only admirers but worshippers.

Napoleon had himself crowned emperor late in 1804, when he was thirty-six. Over the next four years, changes came rapidly. His face became round, his hands pudgy, his hair sparse and silky; he developed a paunch. His sense of grandeur had always been swollen, his temper explosive, but now both seemed to worsen as his self-discipline waned. Intimates feared his ambition and tantrums. Some said he was becoming mad. The crafty Talleyrand began to dissociate himself from what might become a falling star. Although Napoleon was increasingly quarrelsome, he was also sometimes lethargic and unable to concentrate. Carnot, his minister of war, wrote during the Russian campaign: "I no longer know him. He used to be lean, shy, and silent. Now he is fat and garrulous. He is sleepy, and his mind wanders. He, the man of rapid decisions, who resented the proffer of advice, now talks instead of acting, and asks opinions." This was the Napoleon who lost in the clutch at Waterloo.

The change was explained several decades ago as a result of a disordered thyroid gland. A hyperactive thyroid, however, is not enough to send one soaring with Napoleon's drive and genius. And Napoleon's midlife changes poorly fit the picture of myxedema, or thyroid deficiency; furthermore, severe thyroid failure is usually consistent and progressive, while the change in Napoleon was intermittent, incomplete. In the first half of this century, a time of grand discoveries and expectations in endocrinology, hormonal explanations flourished. The thyroid theory is now generally ignored, but more dramatic ones are not.

The most tenacious of these theories rose from an observation by Walter Henry, one of the British doctors who observed Napoleon's autopsy. He wrote that Bonaparte was quite fat and his skin pale, delicate, almost without body hair. "The pubis," he later wrote, "much resembled the mons veneris in women. The muscles of the chest were small, and the shoulders narrow, and the hips wide. The penis and testicles were very small, and the whole genital system seemed to exhibit a physical cause for the absence of sexual desire and chastity which had been stated to have characterised the deceased."

Almost a century later, when there was pioneering excitement about the effects of sex hormones and growth hormones, Henry's words prompted a rediagnosis of Napoleon's midlife changes. Dr. Leonard Guthrie, a London neurologist, wrote in 1913 that the emperor had suffered from Fröhlich's syndrome. This is a deficiency of the pituitary, the "master gland" beneath the brain that regulates much of the rest of the endocrine system, affecting growth, sexuality, and the emotions. In severe form, it arrests body and genital development and causes obesity, mental deterioration, and low physical and mental energy. Other medical historians accepted or elaborated on the idea. The British urological surgeon J. Kemble wrote of Napoleon's "infantile genitals." Dr. A. Cabanes, pointing to the middle-aged Napoleon's corpulence, silky hair, and pudgy hands, pronounced him a pituitary eunuch.

Others went still further. Sir Derrick Dunlop called one account of Napoleon "an admirable description of the youthful eunuchoid or Klinefelter patient." Klinefelter's syndrome is a genetic abnormality that often causes low libido, sterility, and feminized appearance, usually from childhood onward. Today a number of writers continue to suggest that Napoleon soared to greatness on a churning pituitary, burned himself out, and collapsed into a low-pituitary slump of obesity, impotence, crankiness, and lazy dullness. Others have suggested he was driven to his achievements as a compensation for physical, specifically genital, deficiency.

Anyone seeking evidence of Napoleon's "infantile genitals" and "hypogonadism" runs into a thicket of ambiguities. First, Henry's original observation should be read with caution; he seemed to be reaching for an effect. Immediately after emphasizing Napoleon's corpulence, he said that "the whole body was slender and effeminate." Apparently he was pushing the impression of lack of virility every way he could. One wonders whether he allowed for the simple fact that the penis and scrotum may contract against the body after death.

In fact, everyone who stressed Napoleon's shortness and obesity may have exaggerated a bit. Napoleon was over five foot six, probably about average height for a Frenchman in his time. The widespread notion of his shortness comes from inaccurate translation of old French feet, or *pieds de roi;* the French measure of five foot two recorded at autopsy actually translates into five feet six and one half inches in English measure. Napoleon did mock his own unsoldierly plumpness and smooth skin during the sedentary years on St. Helena, saying a woman might envy his arms and breasts. But one cannot be sure that his body changes were abnormal. Many hormonally normal men have little body hair and, in middle age, develop rolls of fat over unexercized chest muscles and the pubis. Even Kemble, who believes Napoleon had a pituitary deficiency, cautions that "the wide hips may have been more apparent than real and due rather to deposition of fat, which in turn produced an appearance of comparative narrowness of shoulders." Napoleon was always described as having small hands; it is hardly startling that they became pudgy when he gained weight. Finally, we should allow that people who expected to meet a titan may have been disappointed to see an average-size man of middle age, going to fat over a slender frame.

Napoleon's "chastity," impotence, or sterility, also alleged as evidence of a pituitary problem, are doubtful.

Napoleon's sex life was a subject of continual gossip while
he lived, chiefly because of Josephine's failure to produce
heirs. He impregnated two other women, felt reassured,
took a second wife, and fathered more with her and with
mistresses. He had a few strong romantic attachments —
to both his wives and to his Polish mistress, Madame Wal-
ewska — but otherwise he seems to have been an abrupt,
peremptory lover. He apparently tended to take sex as he
did food, bolting it during brief breaks from his whirlwind
of work as general and emperor. He did make some re-
marks about his "weakness in the game of love" and com-
mented to intimates about gossip that he might be sterile.
Taken in context, his words suggest at most occasional
psychogenic impotence, especially during his bitter last
years of childless marriage with Josephine. In short, Napoleon seems a clumsy and sporadic lover who lusted more
for power than for women — he himself said, "My mistress is power." But he was hardly impotent or sterile, as
some have seemed intent on proving. There are many
reliable accounts of his sexual encounters with women,
and he recognized in his will not only his legal heirs but
two illegitimate children.

That has not stopped some people, like the blind sages
with the elephant, from seizing one of Napoleon's organs
and arguing tenaciously that it was wanting. The English
writer Shaw Desmond, in his book *Personality and Power,*
asserted that Napoleon, unable to impregnate his second
wife, Maria Luisa of Austria, had her artificially insemi-
nated. He offers no evidence. His predecessor in this theory, a Cuban doctor named Diego Carbonell, suggested
that Napoleon's offspring were actually sired by one of
the emperor's "favorites" — the word seems to have been
chosen for its overtones of homosexuality. Recently Dr.
Frank Richardson, agreeing that Napoleon was sterile,

nominated one of Napoleon's brothers as the royal stud. More later about Richardson, who also maintained that Napoleon was a "bisexual" or "latent homosexual."

The entire range of pituitary theories, which open onto some bizarre avenues, rests on fragmentary and questionable evidence. Even if one could accept the simplistic analogy of that gland, like an engine part, spinning wildly and burning itself out, the fact remains that Napoleon's last years were not the lethargic dumps of a hypopituitary victim. Despite changes, he remained capable at times of stunning energy and brilliance. On Elba he kept busy from dawn till midafternoon and then rode horseback for three hours for refreshment; Colonel Sir Neil Campbell said, "You would think he had discovered the secret of perpetual motion." His dramatic vibrance could revive; facing a regiment sent from Paris to stop his return in 1815, he approached and said, "If one soldier among you wants to kill his emperor, here I am." They lowered their rifles and threw themselves into his service. He went on to raise an army of almost a half-million men, and for the second time threatened to conquer Europe. On the eve of Waterloo, having slept only four hours the previous night, he inspected his advanced posts on horseback in pouring rain, finished work at daybreak, and began the battle. Until the end of his life, he could fascinate and win the loyalty of even his enemies and captors.

Psychology and psychoanalysis have succeeded little better than physical medicine in explaining Napoleon's midlife change and the drive that so many have called demonic. Wilhelm Stekel, one of the great early psychoanalysts, lapsed badly when writing of the conqueror in his book *Impotence in the Male.* He related Napoleon's "hypertrophic ambition" to his "strikingly small, infantile, undersized genitals." The description of swollen ambition is true enough, but the description of Napoleon's genitals is quite a leap from Henry's postmortem observation. A more sensational analysis came in 1973 from Dr. Frank Richardson, in his book *Napoleon: Bisexual Emperor*. He snakes through the most convoluted analyses of Napoleon's psychosexual life and concludes that Bonaparte had "homosexual tendencies" or an "immature homosexual component." (The idea is not his alone; it was suggested a half century earlier by a homosexual writer using the pseudonym Numa Praetorius, who tended to find such tendencies in all famous men.) Richardson goes so far as to place Napoleon at 3 on the Kinsey heterosexual-homosexual scale of 6 — on a basis Kinsey would not have approved. However, Richardson hastens to add that Napoleon never acted out this side of his nature: "It would have been quite alien to Napoleon's character to have stooped to sodomy." With this poorly chosen verb, and references to Napoleon symbolically tweaking subordinates' noses, Richardson settles for declaring the emperor "bisexual," his homosexuality unconscious or latent. In fact, Napoleon was tolerant of homosexuality but scornful of it; his homosexuality seems to be in the eyes of a few beholders eager to find it.

Freud offered more modest analytic attempts, in letters to Arnold Zweig and Thomas Mann. "Napoleon," he wrote to Zweig, "had a tremendous Joseph complex," an unconscious striving to outdo his older brother Lucien. Some studies of birth order do show distinctive personality patterns in first-born, middle, and last-born children, but these are far from universal and don't distinguish Napoleon from millions of other second-born sons. One might make at least as strong a case for the importance of Napoleon's being Corsican, a bit of a second-class citizen to many Frenchmen.

It was Alfred Adler with his concepts of the inferiority complex and overcompensation who did most to fix a psychohistorical version of Napoleon in people's minds. Adler portrayed Napoleon as a pugnacious bantam who made up for his shortness by being overbearing and eventually tyrannical. In addition, he agreed that Napoleon was a typical second child, "rarely able to endure the strict leadership of others . . . inclined to believe, rightly or wrongly, that there is no power in the world which cannot be overthrown." We have already seen that Napoleon was not very short, but we inherit Adler's image of a pint-size bully, and the term "Napoleonic" still falls on people who fail to be passive as well as tall. Grandiose psychotics are shown in comedy acting like Napoleon; as usual, life exceeds art. The great Chilean poet Pablo Neruda noted that in the late thirties, Guatemala was ruled by a military despot named Ubico "with a Napoleon complex. He liked to wear a lock of hair on his forehead, and had his photograph taken a number of times in Bonaparte's famous pose."

Some psychiatrists have called Napoleon a psychopath; others have written of his vast narcissism. He did exhibit grandiosity as his power grew. During the empire he dismissed able advisers and surrounded himself with yesmen. Now, said Chateaubriand, Bonaparte spoke no longer of the people whose revolution he had claimed to represent, but of himself: "I have ordered, I have conquered, I have spoken: my eagles, my crown, my blood, my family, my subjects." Once he had worn a simple uniform amid his splendidly dressed officers. Now he designed his own bejeweled coronation robes, had himself made emperor, adopted the sword and insignia of Charlemagne, and commissioned the famous Canova to sculpt him as a classical demigod, naked except for a fig leaf. In 1808 he pro-

claimed, "God has given me the will and force to overcome all obstacles." In 1811 he predicted that five years
hence he would possess the entire world.

Many writers, such as the famous nineteenth-century
historian Thiers, have said that the change in Napoleon
was entwined with his abuse of power. Author Hugh
L'Estaing speaks of the drive to conquer and dominate as
"the pathology of leadership." Others have called it Caesarism or the malady of power. Dr. Sokoloff, the medical
biographer, argued for a direct connection between the
psychic and physical state; the energy, the tantrums, the
fits of fury and tears, strained and unbalanced Napoleon's
endocrine system; this imbalance worsened the behavior,
and so on in a vicious cycle until the man became a severe
endocrine casualty. Sokoloff notes the same explosive
temperament and nervous symptoms in Caesar and Alexander the Great and says, "Heirs to the same physiological
complex, touched by grandiose visions of Caesarism, all
of them trod the same path, all perished from an excess
of power." The idea is tempting, with its suggestion that
cancerous ambition has a self-limiting flaw. I, too, would
like to believe, as a better writer than Sokoloff put it, that
those who live by the sword shall perish by it. Unfortunately, history offers many despots who died of old age.

We still haven't exhausted the explanations of Napoleon's health, psyche, personality changes, and death. One
minority view is that thin, sallow young Napoleon rose to
power through the frantic exaltation caused by tuberculosis. The disease subsided; then, no longer borne on the
febrile wings of consumption, he became an ordinary,
vulnerable man. Another is that the malaria he allegedly
contracted as a young man permanently blemished his
health. Still another is that he suffered a heart disorder

called the Stokes-Adams syndrome; this idea rose from probably erroneous stories that he had an abnormally slow pulse and could control its pace. These theories, like the allegations of syphilis, secret poisoning, and fatal dysentery and hepatitis, are all possible but have weaknesses. The theories that he had a pituitary disorder and was helped toward death by maltreatment are possible but unproven; I think the balance of evidence is against them. The argument for bilharzia is also unproven, but to me it has a ring of probability. So do a few other ideas.

One suggestion, perhaps too easily dismissed in recent times, is a mild epileptoid condition. Sokoloff linked the malady of power with epilepsy, which apparently afflicted Caesar, Mohammed, and some other famous leaders. Napoleon did have some blackouts and nervous fits; that he had epilepsy was suggested almost a century ago by physical anthropologist Cesare Lombroso. Napoleon's few so-called fits don't match the typical picture of grand mal, and epilepsy hardly seems a prerequisite for power. However, his character and his medical history are consistent with a mild *forme fruste* of epilepsy — his tantrums over small frustrations, which sometimes ended with rolling on the floor or beating his head with his fist, and his lethargy and psychosomatic ills at times of intense activity and stress. However, this remains pure speculation.

There may also be merit in the recurring suggestion that Napoleon died of frustration and boredom. The man who had seized and rattled the world lived cooped up on a tiny island, with nothing to spend his energy on but local gossip and intrigues. If ever there was a man of whom it could be said, "Not working would kill him," it was Napoleon. In 1823, Napoleon's memoirist, Las Cases, asserted Napoleon had really died of frustration and despair. In our time, research in immunology and psychosomatic medicine has shown a link between depression and vulnerability to ills from flu to cancer.

Too few people who write about the change in Napoleon's character give normal aging its due — normal, that is, for a man of Napoleon's character and life experience. I have known and worked with some men of unusual drive and power, and have seen in them some of the same changes. Napoleon, a Machiavellian master of politics and war, grew cynical and cold, finally somewhat jaded. For a while, his power allowed him to insulate himself from the usual checks of daily reality, and to indulge whims without contradiction. He became self-indulgent and pettily tyrannical, like the pasha of a boy's fantasies. And then perhaps he found that one of life's cruelest tricks is giving a man what he most craves. Some of the very powerful suffer fits of weary bleakness. Their ambition is sated. They cannot give up power but now lust for it differently, like men who feel compelled to hold on to lovers they despise. They know the dirty business of power, its brutalities, and can no longer romanticize it. And they become fatalistic from seeing the odd fortunes of the struggle for power. In later life, Napoleon spoke of himself as a fragment of rock hurled through space, a plaything of destiny. The middle-aged Napoleon, who oddly mixed drive and self-indulgence, voracity and lazy mental absence, resembles, on another scale, a number of aging men I have met in luxurious executive suites.

Finally, though, one must not reduce Napoleon to a walking clinic. Despite his ills and vagaries, he had a force that, as historian Herbert Butterfield said, "left a lightning-streak across the pages of history." That energy and impact have sent generations of scholars on his trail, demonstrating the uses and abuses of every approach to history. He continues to resist their efforts to simplify him. He was a despot and a humane reformer; he tore down the ghetto walls of Europe and gave the first demonstration of total war; he was responsible for the first modern dossier-ridden bureaucratic state, but also for a reformist civil code that still underlies much European law; he fostered education and science but hoped to conquer the world over millions of corpses.

Therefore historians have tried to prove a multiplicity of theories over Napoleon's dead body — theories about health, psychology, economics, society, and politics. They have made him a hero or a monster. Some have tried to prove him a plaything of biological forces outside himself. His own Marshal Ney wrote that famine and winter conquered the Grand Army in Russia, and medical historians add that typhus played a part. They are probably partly right, like many who find answers in various parts of Napoleon's body.

Clearly the biohistorian's first job is trying to set the record straight — seeing how likely it is that Napoleon was murdered, whether physical or mental afflictions influenced his judgment. The more complex job is interpreting the facts and probabilities. History is rewritten generation after generation, in an attempt to understand and justify the present and to create a vision of the future. The historic record, of course, is a check on interpretation. The French chauvinist who venerates Napoleon shouldn't be allowed to convince us that the emperor was martyred on St. Helena if that wasn't true. The same rules of evidence must limit the English moralizer who sees Napoleon's illness and defeat as nature's revenge for challenging British imperialism. Psychologists and philosophers should not rest unchallenged when they use wild speculations about Napoleon's mind and body to validate their theoretical hobbyhorses.

If a proctologist prowls in Napoleon's bowels, a urologist in his bladder, a psychoanalyst in his childhood, they may add to the historic record and give interpretation a new dimension. Unfortunately, the view of one specialty risks sounding like intellectual gossip or even an intellectual joke. Justly or not, we tend first to be fascinated, but eventually to grow skeptical, for we suspect that it usually takes much more than constipation, parasites, or sibling rivalry to fully explain a man or event.

The post-postmortem of Napoleon is not over; it may never end. At the present it offers some enlightenment, some interesting possibilities, some foolishness and special pleading — and an example of the limits of medical biography as it has usually been practiced. Its false trails and ambiguities call on future biohistorians to improve their methods and use greater care, imagination, and scope. The following chapter will show how this can be done.

But before leaving Napoleon, we should give a final glance at the question such biography has always raised — whether his itch made the world scratch. The "as if" question in history invites wishful thinking and can support the most eccentric views. It does seem that Napoleon might have won the battles of Borodino and Waterloo had he not been ill. Few people can doubt that Roosevelt's declining health influenced the outcome of the Yalta conference, or that the longevity of Tito and Franco helped shape Europe in this century. The question is the extent of the influence. The answer may depend more on one's convictions, one's view of life, than on hard evidence.

For two millennia, many or most historians have assumed what Thomas Carlyle would defend in his "great man" theory, that extraordinary individuals have guided mankind like tall beacons. During the past century this has become less fashionable. Tolstoy, in *War and Peace,* used Napoleon in his attempt to show that the great shaping force of history is not great leaders or an inspired elite but the power that rises from masses of people — a tide that carries helpless generals and monarchs in its flow. He mentions the "cold" (or whatever ill) that made Napoleon relinquish command at Borodino and rejects the importance of chance in shaping events. Would Napoleon have changed history had he remained fit at Borodino? Patriotic to Russia and to a somewhat mystical view of the power of "the people," Tolstoy said that if this were true, the real savior of Russia was the butler who forgot to give Napoleon watertight boots.

We can each continue in our minds the argument between Carlyle, Tolstoy, and a host of modern determinists from Marxists to doctrinaire psychohistorians. I wish to add an aside from Stendhal. To Tolstoy's comment on the butler saving Russia, Stendhal might have said, with his tongue only halfway in his cheek, "Well, that may be so." There is a war story Stendhal liked to tell, about an officer whose men were wavering in battle, about to break and flee. In desperation, the officer leaped up, waved his saber, and yelled the first impassioned words that entered his mind — something on the order of "Follow me, men! My asshole's as round as a shiny red apple!" Something in this impromptu call touched exactly the right spot in his troops. They followed him in an abandoned charge that won the day.

Why those words? Why that response? What odd wellspring . . . ? Well, most modern university historians might shrug it off and seek the "real" socioeconomic roots of the victory. Great-men theorists would get busy writing about the officer. Tolstoy would probably have said that the troops inspired the officer. But Stendhal would probably smile, skeptical yet knowing, showing his ability to be surprised by life and to remain humble before chance and enigma.

2

Goya sans Syphilis

BIOHISTORY AS DETECTION

WHEN Francisco Goya was forty-six, he suffered an agonizing and mysterious illness. It almost killed him, left him stone deaf, and transformed his personality and art. Until then he had been a skilled, successful, and rather conventional painter. He emerged from his illness a revolutionary giant of Romantic art.

Biographers and doctors playing amateur biohistorian have mechanically repeated the early guess that Goya's malady was syphilis. In retrospect, even a dim-witted medical student should have had doubts. A better explanation finally appeared because a young physician in Dusseldorf happened to be filling a public-health post when the city's bridges were being painted. His rediagnosis of Goya is a fine example of biohistorical detection. And it shows how correcting a medical biography can transcend minor fact-finding and raise questions about the methods of biohistory, occupational and environmental disease, and the natures of personality and creativity.

No definitive biography of Goya yet exists. Like Picasso, his modern counterpart, Goya lived and worked with such ferocious vitality that making the chronicle would be a lifetime's labor. We do know that he was a gilder's son, born in 1746 in Fuendetodos, a dusty village near Saragossa. Saragossa had once been the capital of a proudly independent kingdom of Aragon. Even today, Aragonese pride is notorious. By tradition the Aragonese are tough, brusque, crude, independent, mulish — capable, said Wyndham Lewis, of driving nails into stone walls with their heads and of eating soap to prove it is cheese. Like many stereotypes of regional character, this one is probably an acute half-truth. Certainly Goya fits it. All his life he pushed stubbornly into the wind and spent himself with dark gusto.

As a schoolboy in Saragossa, Goya met two people who would influence and record his life. One was schoolmate Martin Zapater, who also became a painter and exchanged letters with Goya for decades. The other was Francisco Bayeu, a young local artist who would become Goya's brother-in-law and, as painter to the king, help boost Goya into court circles.

Goya showed such artistic precocity that at fourteen he was allowed to help decorate the church in Fuendetodos. He studied painting with Bayeu's old teacher and in 1763 went to Madrid to practice his art. If his arrival there made ripples, they left no lasting mark. After a few years he traveled to Rome, where he presumably more or less made a living as a painter. Legend and inference, more than recorded fact, say that in Madrid and Rome Goya saw a lot of gritty street life, from brawling to love affairs and whoring. Some accounts have the young artist fleeing Saragossa to avoid arrest after a fight, climbing the dome of St. Peter's in Rome, and breaking into a nunnery in pursuit of a lovely novice.

Much of this has been dismissed as legend. True, Zapater recorded that both Fuendetodos and Saragossa remembered young Goya as "restless and turbulent"; he may well have been handy with his fists, even with a knife. And a provincial young artist of Goya's immense energy must have explored every lively alley of such brilliant, bustling capitals as Madrid and Rome. Certainly he always relished depicting the streets, crowds, bullrings, paupers, dandies, fiestas and promenades of Madrilene life. But always Goya's first passion was work; bohemianism *à la* Mürger and Metro-Goldwyn-Mayer was probably as much in the public's imagination as in his life. Still, the picture of Goya as tough, profligate young artist survived, and it was used to support the idea that his crucial illness was syphilis acquired in his youth.

Whatever ambitious young Goya acquired, it wasn't fame. After a few years in Rome, defeated in painting competitions, he returned to Saragossa, worked doggedly at church frescoes, and settled down in marriage with Bayeu's sister Josefa. Then recognition finally flowed to him. He became a popular local portraitist, and with Bayeu's help made connections at the Royal Academy, won commissions from the royal tapestry factory. There were setbacks: Josefa had a number of children who died during or soon after birth; Goya experienced a frustrating run-in with the Church over the orthodoxy of a fresco; in 1778, at age thirty-two, he suffered an illness so severe that he called his recovery a miracle. That sickness, like his allegedly wild youth, would keep turning up in the argument that he had syphilis.

Goya's success kept mounting. He was elected to the Royal Academy, moved to Madrid, found wealthy patrons, and in 1786 was appointed court painter. He bought a carriage, won the right to be called excellency. He began an affair with the mercurial and beautiful young duchess of Alba, whom he would paint as the scandalous *Nude*

Maja. In 1790 he completed a portrait of King Charles IV, who praised and embraced him. The village gilder's son wrote glumly to his old schoolmate Zapater that he had finally hammered his way to "an enviable way of life," but at the cost of wrinkles and a pressing sense of age. He sent Zapater some songs then popular in the night-haunts of Madrid and complained in a letter:

"I go no longer to places where I might hear them, the reason being that I have come to believe I must uphold [a] certain dignity that the human being ought to have — with all of which, as you may well believe, I am not very happy." His self-portraits show a stubborn, stocky man with a pugnacious face, smoldering and weary, caged in expensive collars and hats.

Had Goya's career ended then, he would have survived in passing mention, one of those gifted, popular artists who win laureateships and slightly but distinctly miss greatness. His works, influenced chiefly by Tiepolo, were skilled and lovely, some almost cloyingly sweet. He had a knack for charming pastorals and for street scenes, and his shrewd use of generous white undercoating gave his canvases a striking luminosity. And his portraits did catch his sitters, almost by the scruff of the neck; only in Spain, with its tradition of brutally literal realism, its painted wooden Christs crucified with real nails, would people pay for such blunt accuracy. But by the highest standard, Goya was still an artist of second rank. Perhaps he would have burst free from his fine collars and fat commissions as a predictably successful middle age grew more oppressive. We will never know. Late in 1792, illness thrust change upon him.

The blow was sudden, terrifying. Goya was stricken with dizziness, impaired balance, mental confusion, perhaps hallucinations; convulsions and coma; paralysis of the right side; impaired hearing and speech; relentless ringing in his ears; and most frightful to an artist, partial blindness. All the symptoms point to some overwhelming assault on his nervous system. It seemed a miracle that he survived.

In March 1793, Zapater wrote to the duchess of Alba, "Goya is slightly better but progress is sadly slow. The noises in his head and his deafness have not passed away; however his sight has improved and he no longer has fits of dizziness and can walk up and down stairs without difficulty." It took many more months for most of the symptoms to disappear. Goya returned to his work permanently changed. He remained stone deaf for the rest of his life, and his personality and art began a grand, grim alteration.

The change has struck every critic and biographer as cataclysmic. For instance, John Canaday writes, "Goya's life was split in two near its midpoint by an illness that nearly killed him . . . a new Goya emerged. Goya the humane and bitter social observer, the scourging and despairing delineator of vice and cruelty." All such descriptions pale before the works themselves. There had been occasional hints of the satiric and sinister before Goya's illness, but nothing to prepare one for the despairing savagery of the *Caprices*.

In these etchings, folly, hypocrisy, and nightmare succeed each other. Fops, friars, inquisitors, pedants, are given the heads of beasts. Young dandies court wealthy crones; vacuous, vain ladies mysteriously carry chairs upon their heads; beasts attend beauty, jackass instructs jackass, animal rides man. The brutal poor, the haughty rich, the proud oppressive ranks of the clergy, all flaunt their malice and greed. Creatures with human heads and the bodies of plucked fowl are spitted, roasted alive. Women steal the teeth from hanged men, whores turn away their begging mothers, and shrieking witches wrestle on the winds. A man slumps face down amid winged creatures like bats and cats, and the legend proclaims, "The sleep of reason produces monsters."

Deaf, tortured Goya has been compared to Cruikshank, Callot, and Bosch. But the *Caprices* make Cruikshank seem genteel, Callot whimsical, Bosch studied. They are not products of dream states but nightmares come true, with the unforgiving realism of those peasant Spanish crucifixions. Goya's brutish, agonized figures belong to a special class of art, works that haunt one ever afterward. Like Oedipus with streaming sockets, Lear fumbling with his button, El Greco's Christ writhing flamelike before Toledo, the *Caprices* sear a beholder's mind and inhabit his imagination forever. They are the scream of an artist who could not escape seeing man as clay hopelessly misshapen by a twist in his spirit.

Predictably, enemies recognized their portraits and bristled at the anticlerical tone. Nor did they appreciate the vision, as Baudelaire described it, of "young naked girls adjusting their stockings for the tempting of demons." The Inquisition attacked at once. To protect Goya, the king had to buy the plates, pretend he had commissioned them, and keep the prints out of circulation.

The tough, ambitious Aragonese found ways to survive and thrive. He went on producing portraits, landscapes, and religious works and crowned his career by being named First Painter to the King. Don Manuel Godoy, second in power to the king, took the trouble of learning sign language in order to converse with the deaf artist.

But the grotesque and the anguished had entered Goya's work to stay, and they were fed by private and civil tragedy. His beloved duchess abandoned him, then

died. Spain bled through Napoleon's peninsular campaign
and the long aftermath of civil war, famine, and atrocity.
There is a story that when the revolt broke out against
Napoleon's occupying troops, Goya went at night, blun-
derbuss in one hand and portfolio in the other, to sketch
by torchlight the heaped corpses of slaughtered civilians.
After the French were driven out, a brutal civil war ensued
between liberal and reactionary factions. As usual, in Spain's
sad history, despotism won. Goya spent a decade re-cre-
ating in etchings *The Disasters of War.* They are even more
appalling than the *Caprices* — a panorama not of nightmare but of the realest horrors.

Not one scene in the series shows a military operation.
Shackled civilians kneel before their executioners, and
women await rape beside their murdered children. Singly
and in groups, people are tortured, clubbed, castrated,
garroted, hanged, shot, dragged to death. Their mutilated
torsos and hacked-off heads and limbs festoon the trees
of Spain. The captions say simply "This I saw" and "Why"
and "It is useless to cry out." Man reduces man to a
bleeding side of meat. There is nothing to soften the re-
vulsion and outrage; Goya depicts not history but the most
sickening side of humanity. The *Disasters* are still art's
most desperate cry against the lust for brutality, and against
the wars used to excuse it.

Goya probably finished the *Disasters* a few years before
1820; politics kept them from public view till long after
his death. Meanwhile, his wife Josefa had died, and in
1809 he had suffered another severe illness. Late in 1814
he again faced the Inquisition, this time for having painted,
in the *Nude Maja,* a naked woman, something dared only
once before in Spanish art, by Velásquez. With Leocadia
Weiss, his housekeeper and apparently his mistress, he
retired in 1818 to a house he had bought outside Madrid.

It became known as the Quinta del Sordo, the House of the Deaf Man. On its walls he created the "Black Paintings," ferocious visions in whose presence the deaf old artist ate, slept, and worked.

One shows two men, knee deep in mire, battling in primeval dawn with clubs. Others show a witches' sabbath, Judith wielding a bloody sword, dark figures that seem to have come from a mad Rembrandt. The most fearsome of all is *Saturn Devouring One of His Children* — the god of melancholy, a mad goggle-eyed giant, gnawing at the bloody arm-stump of a man whose head he has already chewed off. The paintings are called black not only for their overwhelming sense of mystery and nihilism but for a few with black backgrounds where barely visible figures lurk. This sinister chorus hovers in the darkness of a painting of 1820, *Self-Portrait with Dr. Arrieta.* The inscription says, "Goya in gratitude to his friend Arrieta for the skill and care with which he saved his life in the acute and dangerous illness suffered at the end of the year 1819, at the age of 73." It shows the artist stricken, head back in exhaustion and pain, one hand clutching the bedsheets, supported by a physician who tries to get him to drink from a glass.

Political reaction kept growing in Spain; no one known for liberal and anticlerical views was safe. In 1824 Goya fled across the Pyrenees to live in Bordeaux. Despite exile, recurrent illness, the isolation of deafness, the other tragedies of his life, he kept growing as an artist to the very end. He experimented in new techniques, worked in every material and genre, and expressed a tremendous range of emotion, from supremely dark, demonic visions to the gently lyric. Past the age of eighty, he created *The Milkmaid of Bordeaux,* a lovely pastoral that capped his early sweet style. Like deaf Beethoven, who was roughly his contemporary, he was a protean artist of relentless force who broke the classical forms he had inherited, to become the first modern master of his art. He died of a stroke in 1828, two weeks after his eighty-second birthday.

Goya was not yet dead when people began trying to explain the sickness that had been his life's watershed. Zapater archly pointed the way in a letter, saying Goya had been led to illness "by his own lack of reflection." Biographers jumped on the implication that youthful whoring or middle-aged affairs in society had left him syphilitic. The idea surely satisfied the sort of prurient moralist who likes to think artists live out his fantasies and pay the price. There was further evidence, some claimed; Josefa Goya allegedly had twenty pregnancies, but only one child survived its early years. Obviously she had caught syphilis from her husband, and it had taken the predictable toll on their progeny.

Syphilis was a safe guess in Zapater's time and even later. Its cause remained unknown, and certain diagnosis impossible, until the turn of this century. It is one of the most complex diseases, its forms myriad, its course unpredictable; an old adage says that to understand syphilis is to understand medicine. Like schizophrenia today, syphilis was long a "wastebasket" diagnosis for a tremendous range of puzzling ills; sometimes it seems that the label has been slapped on half the people in history who didn't die in public executions.

One thing, though, is usually predictable about syphilis. In its final, tertiary stage, untreated syphilis attacks the brain, usually producing disordered thought, vision, hearing, speech, and motion, and eventually paralysis, madness, and death. A typical and pitiful case of tertiary syphilis was Maupassant, who died at forty-four crawling about in an asylum devouring his excrement.

As recently as 1965, an otolaryngologist, or ear-nose-and-throat specialist, named Böhme wrote with confidence that Goya's maladies at thirty-two and forty-six were the second and third stages of syphilis, which caused his deafness. The next year another otolaryngologist, Dr. S. L. Shapiro, pointed at the long lapse between those ailments and suggested a variation on the theme: "basal luetic [syphilitic] meningitis with an accompanying endarteritis of the cerebral vessels. . . . Such a diagnosis would explain the temporary blindness (involvement of the optic nerves), the headaches, the temporary aphasia and paralysis, and the final deafness." In other words, syphilis had paved the way for brain and vascular damage, which led to a stroke at age eighty-two.

It is an odd array of ideas. First: Goya suffered advanced syphilis with brain damage at forty-six. Second: this couldn't be the same ill suffered at thirty-two, because syphilis takes a worse and faster toll. Third: after nearly fatal syphilis, Goya lived another thirty-six remarkably vital years, enjoying all his faculties except his hearing and good humor.

Here, of course, is the flaw in the syphilis theory. No matter how chameleonlike the disease, the odds are very high against someone showing its worst neurological ravages at thirty-two or forty-six and living a vigorous, productive life till eighty-two. And despite hardships, ills, and griefs, Goya was always robust, a blunt weapon of a man whose creative energy kept growing as he aged.

In fact, the only "evidence" for syphilis is Zapater's insinuation. Some historians now say that Josefa had not nineteen pregnancies but four or five; the survival of only one of that number wasn't unusual in Goya's day. Interestingly, the picture of Goya as suffering, sinful artist has had support from analogy — to Beethoven, whose deafness was also alleged by some to have resulted from syphilis. That case is equally flimsy; there is at least as good a case that Beethoven was a victim of nerve deafness.

Clinging to the theory that Goya's midlife crisis of health and personality was syphilis demands either ignorance or devout attachment to the idea. Why have so many biographers and doctors stood by it? The only explanation is the Law of Repetition. Our second venture in biohistory demands a few meanders, and this one is essential, for we will meet this law often as we proceed.

The Law of Repetition was first pointed out to me by one of my professors. I decided to study a poet who is always represented in anthologies by the same single poem. I read his complete works, found a dozen poems just as fine, and asked in my term paper why anthologists stuck to the same one. My teacher responded in the margin, "Because most anthologists only bother to read other anthologists."

The law of lazy repetition lies behind much inherited error, and it flourishes when specialists reach into other specialties. A historian, trained to question even firsthand accounts with a trial lawyer's skepticism, may worshipfully buy what any doctor says on a medical point. A doctor, trained to demand laboratory proofs, may regurgitate the silliest historical summary he finds because its author had an advanced degree. Each knows the complex rigors of his own field; yet his very respect for expertise may make him credulous in other fields. Instead of rechecking and seeking verifications, he repeats the first "authority" he reads or even off-the-cuff opinions and secondhand summaries.

Zapater's hint that Goya might have had syphilis appealed to moralism, fantasy, and drama. It handily answered a biographical puzzle. Historian and doctor alike failed to seek a second opinion, and the patient was past protest.

But if not syphilis, what? Some ear-nose-and-throat specialists have guessed otosclerosis or Menière's syndrome; either might account for Goya's deafness and vertigo, but for little else. Some psychiatrists have guessed schizophrenic or depressive psychosis, which explain even less and rests on as little evidence. Each specialist reaches for his part of the elephant; the podiatrists and proctologists remain to be heard from.

One recent guess does deserve serious attention, because it is based on both clinical experience and some historical thought. It was made in 1962 by Dr. Terence Cawthorne of England, who pointed to a malady as rare as it is untripping on the tongue — the Vogt-Koyanagi syndrome.

Cawthorne reminds us of an incident in Goya's life. Not long before his crucial sickness, he rode over the Sierra Morena mountains in the duchess of Alba's carriage, and in a wild gale the axle broke. Goya called for tools and helped make the repair; as a result, he suffered a fever. Some details and the precise date have been disputed, but the event and approximate time are likely enough.

Cawthorne dismisses syphilis, suggests a very different sort of illness, and cries Eureka: "Exposure to cold and over-exertion when trying to mend the axle . . . have been put forward as exciting causes of the illness; but of course in everybody's mind, both at that time and since, was [syphilis]. Nevertheless, the fact that he recovered . . . suggests that this was a sudden episode without any progressive spread of the disease as would be expected in the later stages of syphilis, either of the nervous or cardio-vascular system. It is much more likely to have been a curious syndrome in which temporary inflammation of the uveal tract is associated with permanent deafness. . . . To the full-blown syndrome are attached the names of Vogt and Koyanagi, and I have seen 5 patients exhibiting all or most of the features of this disorder."

The idea came to Cawthorne when he treated a man of forty-six, exactly Goya's age when he fell ill. He had suddenly been attacked by deafness, severe giddiness, and eye inflammation. Within two months his eyes had cleared, but he didn't regain his hearing or balance. Cawthorne had his diagnosis confirmed by a colleague. "I believe," he concluded, "that it was the syndrome from which Goya suffered."

Certainly it fits Goya much better than syphilis. This syndrome, still little understood, is probably caused by a virus and sometimes leaves its victims permanently deaf. As for the change in personality, Cawthorne says it could have resulted from the illness, from deafness, or from having witnessed the ghastly Peninsular War. He compares Goya to Swift, "who, a century earlier, was subject to recurring bouts of severe deafness and giddiness due to Menière's disease. . . . Both were sociable, lively, and popular in high society. Each was robbed of his hearing in middle life, and being forced into loneliness each became a prey to morbid thoughts which may well have affected his artistic output."

Rare, poorly understood viral disease? Possibly, but another diagnosis seems even better, and it is based on a longer, finer sifting of evidence on Goya's health, personality, and art. In fact, it is receiving more confirmation each year from such distant sources as studies of poisoned slum children and industrial workers. The author of this theory, like Cawthorne, had a flash of recognition when he compared Goya's symptoms to those of his own patients. That story goes back more than fifty years.

In the early 1930s, Dr. William Niederland was serving his medical residence in Dusseldorf. To pick up some extra money he filled a public-health post and received as patients the workers who were scraping and repainting the city's bridges. Exposed to large amounts of lead in the paint they breathed and handled, they suffered from plumbism, or lead poisoning. Many showed acute encephalopathy, or damage to the brain. Niederland's work with the bridge painters got him deeply involved in the study of lead poisoning, and he wrote a report on it as an environmental and industrial problem for the health organization of the League of Nations.

Dr. Niederland began to add psychiatric training to his knowledge of physical medicine. Then crisis interrupted his life. A Jew, he had to leave Nazi Germany. In the United States he completed his psychoanalytic training and began private practice in New York City. Because of his love of art, many creative artists eventually entered his office, especially painters and sculptors. Over the years, Niederland added another dimension to his work; besides his background in physical medicine, industrial medicine, and psychoanalysis, he had an abiding interest not only in art but in history. He wrote a fascinating psychoanalytic study of the life, work, and personality of Heinrich Schliemann, the passionate and erratic nineteenth-century adventurer who defied conventional wisdom, sought and discovered the ruins of Troy, and helped found the science of archaeology.

Around 1960, Niederland's many specialties and interests focused together on the case of an artist whose work he deeply loved. Reading accounts of Goya's illness, he immediately thought of the bridge painters he had treated thirty years earlier in Dusseldorf. The clinical match seemed perfect, the standard syphilis diagnosis facile and unlikely.

"The more I looked," he said to me when we discussed his work, "the less basis I saw for the syphilis argument, and the more I saw a need to understand the crucial break in the artist's personality after his illness. It seemed to me a puzzle of tremendous scientific and artistic importance. After all, look at Goya's earlier works — rococo, almost overly gentle. After the illness a new artist emerged who was embittered, almost cruel. Why? How? That interested me so much that I really got to work. I had to examine not only the possibility of lead poisoning as a diagnosis but historical material to back it up."

That is precisely where Niederland differed from so many medical biographers. Dissatisfied by the lack of an authoritative life of the artist, he did his own research, anticipating questions and arguments against his theory. Too many physicians trying historical diagnosis have picked up one or two books and accepted the historical specialists' first word as the last word.

"I knew," he said, "that there was a wealth of unpublished material about Goya in the archives of the Prado, in Madrid — thousands of items in many languages. I could read documents in several languages other than Spanish, and my wife's Spanish is perfect. We made several trips to Spain over several years."

His years of digging paid off richly in confirming details, and they demanded following byways as interesting as the main road. They ranged from reconstructing Goya's work habits and palette to restudying lead poisoning, which is again the subject of intensive research as one of man's most widespread and pernicious environmental diseases.

Lead poisoning, like syphilis, is difficult to diagnose because its symptoms and severity vary so much. Yet it was one of the first diseases clearly described in medical history. The Egyptians used lead, and plumbism was clearly described by the Greek physician and poet Nicander more than two thousand years ago. The Roman Vitruvius, in his great treatise on architecture, warned against using lead pipes for conducting drinking water, and Pliny mentioned poisoning caused by the lead in pottery glazes, food additives, and storage vessels. (The women of Athens and Rome also used white lead — the lead compound basic to white paint well into this century — as a cosmetic.) The Greeks and Romans did not know that lead poisons not only by being swallowed and inhaled (as dust or in volatile compounds) but by being absorbed through unbroken skin. Nevertheless, they recognized the signs of chronic plumbism: kidney damage, swollen abdomen, the ashen skin of anemia, a "dropped" or limp wrist, and weak limbs.

A little more was observed during the late Middle Ages, when an increase of mining and smelting brought renewed interest in the diseases of metal workers. Then in 1700 Bernardino Ramazzini, a Venetian physician, produced his *Diseases of Workers,* the founding classic of occupational and industrial medicine; it contained a clearer, more detailed picture of lead poisoning than ever before. In 1839 the French physician Tanquerel des Planches described lead neuropathy, the terrible attack on the central nervous system that often comes with acute plumbism. Categorizing by symptoms, he named four forms, characterized by delirium, coma, convulsions, or a combination of the three. Because this fearsome malady often causes deep depression, des Planches called it encephalopathia saturnina, invoking the god of melancholy Goya portrayed in the most gruesome of the Black Paintings.

The descriptions of Ramazzini and des Planches, Goya's recorded symptoms, the sufferings of the bridge painters of Dusseldorf, all matched: paralysis of the limbs, tremor, coma, delirium, transient blindness, mental confusion, depression, paranoid thinking, vertigo. Two of the Dusseldorf painters had recurring depression for a year, as Goya did. After the crisis passed, they still suffered vertigo, impaired sight and hearing, and personality changes. There was the same surprising recovery from devastating illness; just as Goya returned from death's door, one Dusseldorf painter recovered from total paralysis of one side, epileptoid seizures, disorientation, and paranoia. Sickness had meant no contact with lead-base paints; when the painters returned to their trade, many suffered an onslaught of the same symptoms. None of the Dusseldorf patients showed total, permanent deafness, but otherwise they matched Goya symptom for symptom.

The case was dramatic, suggestive; here many medical biographers would have stopped in triumph. Niederland still considered the case circumstantial, for a logical objection lay unanswered. How do we know that Goya was exposed to as much lead as the Dusseldorf workers, enough to bring a visitation from Saturn on leaden wings?

A partial answer lay in Ramazzini's classic of 1700. Today highly toxic lead compounds are banned in the manufacture of paint. But in Ramazzini's day, artists' materials were so toxic that an entire chapter was given to their ills, and most of that chapter to the symptoms of lead and mercury poisoning (mercury was also used widely in pigments and produces many of the same effects). Ramazzini wrote that like miners and potters,

"Painters are attacked by various ailments such as palsy of the limbs, cachexia, blackened teeth, unhealthy complexions, melancholia and loss of the sense of smell. It very seldom happens that painters look florid or healthy . . . [the most immediate cause is] the materials of the colors they handle and smell constantly, such as red lead, cinnabar [containing mercury], white lead . . . and

the numerous pigments made of various mineral substances. . . . Moreover, painters when at work wear dirty
clothes smeared with paint, so that their mouths and noses
inevitably breathe tainted air. . . .

"Fernel illustrates this and records a rather curious case
of a painter of Anjou who was seized first with palsy of
the fingers and hands, later with spasms of these parts,
and the arm too was similarly affected; the disorder next
attacked his feet . . . Fernel goes on to say that, since this
painter was in the habit of squeezing the color from his
brush with his fingers and worse still was imprudent and
rash enough to suck it, it is probable that the cinnabar
was carried from the fingers to the brain by direct communication and so to the whole nervous system. . . . This,
then, and no other is the explanation of the cachetic condition of painters, their unhealthy coloring and the melancholic fits to which most of them are subject."

To this tempting evidence a question must be put: were
painters of Goya's times, a century later, still victims of
their paints? Niederland learned that research on this already existed. In 1934 the German art historian Max Doerner, in his book *The Materials of the Artist and Their Use
in Painting,* had stated that Goya used cinnabar and that
most of his paintings were done over primings of toxic
lead white. In 1941 another scholar, F. Schmid, recreated
Goya's palette and concluded that the pigment Goya used
most was lead white. The harmless pigments now in common use — red without mercury, white based on titanium
and zinc — were not developed till a half century after
Goya's death. And in Goya's day, before factory-made
paints, an artist had to grind and mix his own pigments.

Now Niederland had no doubts. Goya, he wrote, had
been in "frequent and direct contact with the toxic lead
compound which is essentially basic carbonate of lead,

namely, 2 $PbCO_3$, $Pb(OH)_2$. Grinding this poisonous compound into paint is particularly hazardous, since it facilitates inhalation or ingestion by manual handling." Goya's palette also included toxic lead chromate, and mercury-base pigments just as poisonous as lead; both can cause similar symptoms.

Again, the facile biohistorical detective would rejoice and stop. Again Niederland probed his theory for weak spots, found one, and sought evidence. Why should Goya have suffered so acutely from lead poisoning, when many other painters did not? The answer lay in further details about Goya's artistic techniques.

First, Goya used lead white massively in both his primings and his painting. No color was as important to him as the lead white that gave many of his works their famous mother-of-pearl luminosity. Niederland, as an example, points to the famous large canvas called *Winter,* "with its 'leaden' sky, landscapes and figures. Many of Goya's canvases have an iridescent, sparkling quality, with almost infinite gradations of white, whitish gray, and twilight gray."

Second, Goya was amazingly prolific and probably the fastest great portraitist in history. He is said to have finished the portrait of his wife that hangs in the Prado in one hour; a large picture of King Fernando in one or two sessions; a portrait of the Infante Don Luis in a single morning. He did this not only because of his extraordinary gifts but because he worked as Picasso did — like a fountain, an eruption, a tide. Théophile Gautier, in his book *Wanderings in Spain,* gathered anecdotes and concluded:

"What a strange painter, what a singular genius was Goya! . . . His method of painting was as eccentric as his talent. He scooped his color out of tubs, applied it with sponges, mops, rags, anything which he could lay his hands on. He trowelled and slapped his colors on like a bricklayer, giving characteristic touches with a stroke of his thumb. In this extemporary way he covered thirty feet or so of wall in a couple of days. . . ."

So there was Goya, grinding toxic lead and mercury pigments and mixing them with solvents, splashing and mopping his paints, handling them constantly, doubtless splattering himself and his clothes — in short, spending his life in a storm of flying paint. Niederland estimated that through inhalation alone Goya probably absorbed two or three times as much lead as most painters, most of whom, says Ramazzini, were chronically lead-poisoned. Some of Goya's self-portraits seem to show the pallor typical of lead poisoning, and one may suggest the typical distortion of the hands.

Now, armed with interlocking evidence from medical, historical, and artistic sources, Niederland was ready to review past diagnoses. Syphilis, of course, was least likely. Almost as unlikely were speculations by some recent psychiatrists that Goya's personality, art, or health had been shaped by manic-depressive psychosis, involutional depression, or schizophrenic psychosis associated with deafness. Despite the old saw relating genius and madness, and despite some schizophrenics' alleged creativity, most schizophrenic art lacks overall organization or shows compulsively repeated themes. No psychotic has produced the range and depth of art that came from Goya during the second half of his life. In fact, his productivity, versatility, and range of emotions are powerful evidence against schizophrenia and other severe mental ills.

In 1972, after more than a decade of detection, Niederland's paper "Goya's Illness" appeared in the *New York State Journal of Medicine.* It reviewed Goya's life, work, and medical history, making the case for lead poisoning. It pointed out that in 1778, at thirty-two, Goya suffered a nearly fatal illness but fully recovered. Between 1778 and 1781 he apparently experienced depression so deep that it sometimes kept him from his work. In 1792–93 occurred the grave illness, attacking the nervous system, that left him deaf. Other, undescribed illnesses occurred around 1809, 1820, and perhaps later. Each of these illnesses, from age thirty-two till almost eighty, kept Goya away from his paints — which, as the bridge painters of Dusseldorf showed, allows the victim's body level of lead to drop, bringing a return of good health until lead reaccumulates.

Each of Goya's symptoms can be explained by lead and other heavy-metal poisoning. And Niederland reinterprets the words that led to the misdiagnosis of syphilis, Zapater's phrase about "lack of reflection." As Niederland said to me, expanding on his essay, "Zapater remained a modest civil servant in the provincial capital of Saragossa while his old school chum became first painter of the royal court in Madrid. The friendship eventually chilled because of that. Zapater may well be suspected of a sort of sibling rivalry. Or, if you prefer, pomposity growing from envy." Niederland also notes that Goya's nineteen stillborn and miscarried children are quite probably a myth; even if they were not, plumbism would explain them. Lead poisoning causes above-average rates of abortion, stillbirth, and fetal damage.

The neurological damage of lead poisoning may not only cause depression but bring lasting personality change. Furthermore, Niederland agrees with other researchers that Goya's case fits a pattern familiar to those who work with the deaf. "Adults who have been left stone deaf," says Niederland, "often show embitterment and a tendency to depression. There is also often a tinge of aggressive paranoia; a deaf person sees others talk and suspects they're talking about him. Look at the face of deaf Beethoven, and you see a resemblance to Goya's expression in the self-portraits, depressed and bitter. Many people, once gentle, become unbearable in the family setting after deafness strikes."

True, Niederland wrote in his paper, Goya's change wasn't utterly abrupt; there were notes of the melancholy, grotesque, and sinister in some of his early work. Yet Goya did emerge from his illness a different person and a different artist. Did the effects of lead poisoning and deafness build on something latent in the personality? Logically one would suspect that the disease unlocked rather than created Goya's despairing outlook. "But now," Niederland says, "that logic does not satisfy me. Despite any premorbid personality structure, the investigation is not complete. We've made a step toward understanding the riddle of his personality break, but we still must answer a final question. Why did he undergo this change rather than some other?"

Niederland continues his research. Meanwhile, evidence has kept appearing that supports his theory of lead poisoning. For decades plumbism was considered a problem of the past, controlled by public-health measures in mining, manufacture, and consumer protection. In the late 1950s and early 1960s, interest rapidly resumed. Slum children were eating lead, and people all around the world were breathing it in.

Children who lived in dilapidated houses with cracked or peeling lead-base paint were chewing paint chips and suffering from acute plumbism, including encephalopathy. Lead poisoning through pica — the tendency of small children to chew and eat nonfoods such as clay and paint chips — became the object of massive public information campaigns and screening programs. This childhood lead poisoning wasn't new, but it often went unidentified because of such puzzling, multiple symptoms as vomiting, hyperactivity, dizziness, and headaches. Encephalopathy can leave permanent damage from small learning deficits to retardation, epilepsy, cerebral palsy, and blindness. According to one estimate nearly 200,000 children a year suffer permanent brain damage or retardation because of lead poisoning. A leading researcher in the field, J. Julian Chisholm, Jr., points out:

"The symptoms of even acute encephalopathy are nonspecific, resembling those of brain abscesses and tumors and of viral and bacterial infections of the brain. Diagnosis depends first of all on a high level of suspicion. To make a positive diagnosis it is necessary to show high lead absorption as well as the adverse effects of lead."

There has also been growing conviction that lead alkyl, used for almost a half century as an anti-knock gasoline additive, has become a worldwide environmental pollutant through auto exhaust. Few researchers doubt that urban dwellers now carry at least a hundred times the body burden of lead they would bear under nonindustrial conditions.

Further research on lead poisoning has produced facts that buttress Niederland's diagnosis of Goya:

— When lead is ingested, less than 10 percent is absorbed by the intestines; the rest is excreted through the bowel. But lead inhaled as dust or a volatile compound is far more dangerous; some 30–60 percent is retained by the body. There is no doubt that Goya's grinding and mixing of pigments exposed him to extreme danger.

— Much of the lead absorbed by the body may be stored in the bones, which allow a temporarily harmless reservoir

to exist without causing illness. At some critical point, the
bones can hold no more, and the excess enters such soft
tissues as the kidneys, liver, aorta, and brain, producing
acute symptoms. Therefore one can be exposed to lead
for a long period and suddenly show symptoms of acute
poisoning.

— Illness or trauma can precipitate lead stored in the
bones. Someone with Goya's lead level, afflicted with fever,
illness, a fracture, an apparently unrelated change in body
chemistry or living conditions, could suffer the abrupt trig-
gering of acute lead poisoning.

We will never be able to assay Goya's blood, bones, or
aorta for lead, so we will never identify his illness beyond
a doubt. Perhaps Cawthorne was right about the Vogt-
Koyanagi syndrome. But remember Chisholm's caution
that lead encephalopathy resembles viral brain infections
and many other ills: "Diagnosis depends first of all on a
high level of suspicion." And recall that many illnesses
can activate poisonous lead harmlessly stored in the bones.
Most important, Niederland's diagnosis invites assent because it satisfies a rule we must usually abide by in the
complex detection of biohistory, the law of parsimony.
We must provisionally accept the most economical answer
to a problem. That is, we must choose the answer that
accounts for the most facts in the most probable way. Goya
may have even suffered from some disease still undefined
by science, but for the moment, lead encephalopathy is
the most likely malady.

Dr. Niederland's scrupulous, sophisticated, multidisci-
plinary detective work is a model of the sort i.eeded in
biohistory. Niederland is now pursuing the break in Goya's
personality, the radical change in his art. Here he touches
one of the recurrent, endlessly intriguing questions of

biohistory, the relationship between states of the body and states of the mind. Lead encephalopathy, deafness, hormonal changes, alterations of body chemistry, even diet and climate, can affect the personality. How that happens is one of the misty frontiers of science today. It is one of the questions we must consider next.

3

What Ailed Poor Poe?

THE BIOHISTORIAN AS SKEPTIC

𝐼N 1849, Edgar Allan Poe was found dying in a Baltimore street, victim of some malady that experts still debate. Ever since, his name has evoked a somber, sickly figure haunting American literature. Critics remain a hung jury; to some he is a jingling crowd-pleaser, to others America's most original writer. Few men have drawn so many gossips, scholars, and psychohistorians. They have called him everything from a mad drunkard to a victim of his nation's philistinism. Researchers have found the key to his life, work, and death in alcoholism, opium addiction, epilepsy, brain damage, diabetes, childhood trauma, vague hereditary horrors, and the madness called kin to genius There is probably a theory for each of his forty years.

Studies of Poe's ills of body and mind show why the biohistorian must remain a perennial skeptic, alert to every rustle of faddism in the intellectual landscape. His case became a testing ground for the favorite theories of each generation after his death; in fact, their successive diagnoses present a capsule history of social attitudes and scientific fashions over a century and a half. We suggest still another theory. But since so many people have immersed themselves in Poe lore, shouted Eureka, and invented a square wheel, the biohistorian must be sure that he and his contemporaries aren't doing it again.

On one point there is no argument: Poe's life was a series of lost loves and blasted hopes. His paternal grandfather, David Poe, had been an honorary general in the Revolution; his father, David Poe, Jr., disappointed his family by marrying an actress and joining her as a nomadic player. Erratic, ill-tempered, probably a drinker, he disappeared from history when he apparently deserted his pretty, talented wife Elizabeth, who was pregnant with their third child and sick with consumption. Elizabeth struggled to support herself and the children, but late in 1811, twenty-four years old and destitute, she died in a rented room in Richmond. General Poe had taken in her oldest child, William; one Richmond matron took the infant Rosalie, and another took Edgar, who was almost three. Thus Edgar ended up in the home of Scots tobacco merchant John Allan and his wife Frances. There he first received the best possible upbringing, and later the unhappiest.

Though stubborn and frugal, John Allan could be good humored, and he was fond of Edgar. His wife doted on the boy, and he on her. Business took the Allans to England from 1815 to 1820, and there Edgar began his education in good boarding schools. Back in Richmond at eleven, he continued his schooling with the sons of wealthy planters. There was nothing gloomy or sickly about him. He was slender but athletic, a fine swimmer and boxer; teachers and friends would recall him as bright, cheerful, a natural leader. Still, he kept to himself outside school; few friends ever saw his home or stepparents. Amid the antebellum plantocracy, he was aware of being the orphan of actors, raised but not adopted by an ambitious mer-

chant. Some of his friends went on to the University of
Virginia, and Edgar joined them there for part of a year.
From then on, his life often seemed a struggle against
sliding downhill.

The so-called gentlemen of Virginia spent less time at
books than drinking, dueling, and gambling. Personable
but scholarly, Edgar kept busy creating poems of preco-
cious brilliance. Unfortunately, John Allan had sent him
off without enough money for books, food, and lodging.
Edgar tried to win the difference at cards, lost, and had
to write home for help. Allan refused. Edgar's letters
ranged from imploring to bitter, Allan's from stony to
harsh. Finally Edgar had to leave school, shamed by debts
and dunned by creditors. He returned home to find that
he and Allan were adversaries.

The rift still leads biographers to pyrotechnics of inference. Perhaps the up-from-under merchant, having sent
his ward to the best schools in England and Virginia,
couldn't comprehend the brilliant young gentleman who
emerged. More important, perhaps, was Edgar's devotion
to Mrs. Allan. Now she was ailing, and John Allan probably blamed her for his lack of natural heirs. He had
fathered several illegitimate children whose existence was
public knowledge. Edgar probably knew of them, may
even have confronted Allan and taken Mrs. Allan's side.
In any case, he must have felt the stability of his foster
home fading, and he suffered other losses as well. At
fifteen he had experienced his first romantic passion, for
Jane Stannard, the mother of one of his friends. He wor-
shipped this warm woman and visited her when he was
unhappy at home. Before long she died of brain cancer,
and though it may be apocryphal that he visited her grave
every night, he grieved deeply and later wrote "To Helen"
in her memory. A year later he fell in love with a girl

named Elvira Royster and hoped to marry her. When he returned from the university, he found her engaged to an older man with better prospects, perhaps through the machinations of her father and Mr. Allan. And now, with Mrs. Allan ill, his "Dear Pa" was impatiently begetting bastards about town.

Whatever the reasons, John Allan apparently decided to drive Edgar from his heart and home. He did it systematically, refusing him enough money to live on and then attacking him as a wastrel. At last they quarreled violently, and early in 1827 Edgar left home for good. Probably fearing debtors prison, he fled to Boston and enlisted in the army as Edgar G. Perry.

Poe continued to write, and that summer a small edition of his poems appeared; there were few sales and no reviews. At least the army thought well of him; after a year and a half he rose to sergeant major, the highest noncommissioned rank. With the rest of a five-year enlistment yawning before him, he begged Allan for help so that he could hire a substitute to finish his hitch and apply to West Point. First Allan refused, but in February 1829, Mrs. Allan died, the two men had a lukewarm reconciliation, and Allan enabled Edgar to leave the ranks.

Late that year, when Edgar was still twenty, his second book of poems appeared, and it brought a small taste of recognition. Then he went on to West Point, in a final attempt to make peace with Allan and prepare for a career. As at Virginia, he didn't receive enough money even for books. For a while he scraped along — as always, writing poetry and reading voraciously in literature, languages, and science. Eventually Allan's stinginess drove him to the wall, and they had another epistolary brawl, Edgar pained and bitter, Allan frosty and accusing. This time Allan disowned him. In an embarrassment of debts,

Edgar could only deliberately neglect his duties until a sympathetic superior freed him with a dishonorable discharge.

Again Edgar was broke and on his own. For a while he stayed in Manhattan, trying in vain to join the Polish army. His poems appeared in a revised second edition and won a few notices, but the young author of "To Helen" and "The City in the Sea" couldn't rise from destitution to penury. He had only one haven, the relatives he'd discovered two years earlier in Baltimore. There, crowded together in poverty, were General Poe's sick old widow, Edgar's brother William, his widowed aunt Maria Clemm, and her seven-year-old daughter Virginia. Edgar had never fully belonged anywhere. The Baltimore household were blood kin, and to them he now turned.

Soon after Edgar joined them, his brother died, probably of illness and drink; then his grandmother went, and with her the little pension that had kept the family from hunger. Now Edgar was the only support for Mrs. Clemm and Virginia. In those days of low fees and no copyright laws, it was all but impossible to make a living writing, but that was the only thing Poe knew, so he tried. He turned his hand to book reviews, satiric literary sketches, and burlesques of the fantastic Gothic horror stories then so popular. His work was published for a few dollars here, five dollars there, and he poured out more.

Though poor and overworked during his four years in Baltimore, Poe finally had a family unreservedly his own. He devoted himself to the motherly Mrs. Clemm and bright, pretty Virginia — Muddy and Sissy he called them. People described him as energetic, industrious, sometimes grave, but often lively and cheerful. Although he always wore the same threadbare black coat buttoned to the chin, he gave the impression of a gentleman, and of one somehow above the ordinary. He was striking if not quite hand-some, five feet eight inches tall, with brown hair and eyes that seemed gray or hazel with the light. His voice was melodious, his speech precise, his manner easy yet courtly, and he bore himself with a soldier's erectness.

In 1835, when Poe was offered a trial job on *The Southern Literary Messenger* in Richmond, he moved there and sent money to the Clemms from his pitiful salary. Then a cousin, Neilson Poe, offered to take in and support thir-teen-year-old Virginia. If Edgar hadn't realized it before, he did now: little Sissy was blossoming, and he'd been falling in love with her. And he was about to lose both her and the Clemm household. He crashed into a terrifying depression, drank, and almost lost his job. In panic he wrote to Mrs. Clemm, begging her to let Virginia decide whether to marry him or to live with Neilson Poe. To Virginia he wrote, "My love, my own sweetest Sissy, my darling little wifey, think well before you break the heart of your cousin Eddy."

His desperate, abject love won over the girl and her mother; marriage was agreed on, and they moved to Rich-mond. His melancholy lifted, he stopped drinking, and he was made an editor of the *Messenger* on condition that he not drink again. The next spring, Edgar and Virginia mar-ried. He was twenty-seven, she not quite fourteen. Biog-raphers would weave intricate theories about Poe's "child bride" and the start of his drinking under pressure. At the time, Poe was busy just trying to survive.

For a year and a half at the *Messenger,* Poe worked six or seven days a week and filled the pages with his own poems, tales, reviews, and journalism. He turned out to be an excellent editor, with a shrewd eye for feature sub-jects; the magazine's circulation grew from 500 to 3,500, and it won a national reputation. The owner, asserting his authority and ego, fired the man who had the task but neither the pay nor title of editor, and spread tales that the reason was drunkenness. Correspondence and memoirs suggest that although Poe did drink occasionally, he was fired chiefly for excellence.

The Poes moved to New York, and Edgar struggled to establish a career there, but it was a time of financial panic, with little to be made from magazines. After a frustrating year and a half, they went to Philadelphia, where for six years Poe slaved at poetry, hack writing, editing, anything he could find. His tales appeared in book form but found few buyers, and his bitter experience at the *Messenger* was repeated twice. First, at *Gentleman's Magazine,* the owner postured as editor while Poe built circulation. When Poe refused to tone down some reviews, they quarreled and parted ways; with the old *Messenger* incident as ammunition, the owner spitefully claimed Poe had again been fired for drinking. Poe wanted to start his own magazine and sought backers in vain for the rest of his life. Meanwhile, he took a job at *Graham's Magazine.* There he published Lowell and Longfellow, raised the subscription list from 5,500 to almost 40,000, and contributed his own work by the sheaf. He resigned in May 1842, disgusted by his low salary and the owner's bland policy.

In Philadelphia, Poe earned a national reputation as an editor and reviewer, but he was neither prosperous nor popular. He rarely failed to praise the best writers of his day, but in literary quarrels he sometimes turned petty and caustic, and could be acid toward books he thought shoddy. He seemed intent, recalled his boss George Graham, not on reforming error but exterminating it. That has never won favor in commercial publishing or literary politics. On balance, Poe was a first-rate if waspish critic who erred on the side of gallantry toward mediocre women poets. In a time of ferocious cliques and puffery, he made many enemies with access to print, and some never ceased pursuing him.

He especially had to fight gossip that he was a drunk. G. B. Shaw exaggerated in saying that Poe imbibed less in his whole life than the average American does in six months, but Poe never did drink regularly. His habits were generally disciplined and abstemious, and people who knew him well said that they saw him drink nothing stronger than coffee for months or years at a time. Nathaniel Willis, like other contemporaries of Poe, recorded that "with a *single* glass of wine, his whole nature was reversed. . . ." Apparently this happened rarely until his last years, but with memorable effects. When he was accused for the second time of having been fired for drinking, he wrote in explanation to a physician friend that in Richmond he had given way, "at long intervals, to the temptation held out on all sides by the spirit of Southern conviviality. My sensitive temperament could not stand an excitement which was an everyday matter to my companions." But he denied that he had ever been habitually drunk, and had been soused only once in the past four years.

Even if we allow that he may have been retouching his portrait a bit, we must accept the basic picture, confirmed by many witnesses. The problem was that Poe had an abnormally low tolerance for alcohol, and even one drink devastated his mind and body. He quickly became wildly excited, voluble, sometimes pugnacious, and for days afterward felt sick and humiliated. He lived under terrible pressures in a hard-drinking society, but knowing what alcohol did to him, he sought its instant euphoria only when he felt he was drowning. Unfortunately, that happened more often with the years, and a drunk Poe was memorably different from a sober Poe — especially to resentful bosses and rivals.

Early in 1842, such problems abruptly became petty. Virginia burst a blood vessel while singing at the piano, and for two weeks she hung at the edge of death. It was tuberculosis. Her illness dragged on for five years, while Poe alternated between hope and the dread that death would take her as it had his mother, stepmother, and Mrs. Stannard. Editor George Graham said that Poe's love for Virginia was "a sort of rapturous worship," and he hovered over her with "all the fond fear and anxiety of a mother with her first-born child, her slightest cough causing him a shudder, a heart-chill that was visible."

She needed food, medicine, a warm home. Poe wrote furiously. He even sought a government job in Washington, but he drank in the clutch, went for interviews in a voluble high, and ruined his chances. In 1844 he again put his hopes in a literary career in New York. This time, because of Virginia's health, he took a cottage in Fordham, then a village miles north of Manhattan. Early in 1845 luck seemed to arrive. "The Raven" appeared in a New York newspaper and made him famous. ("The Gold Bug" had become rather popular a couple of years earlier, but as Poe said, "the bird beat the bug all hollow.") His stories and poems soon appeared again in book form and sold moderately well, and he gained recognition in England and France.

Still, though Poe often worked sixteen hours a day as writer, editor, and lecturer, he remained desperately poor. He wrote that he sometimes felt sunk in madness or a terrible dream, "but indeed I have had abundant reason to be so." He became an editorial assistant on a New York magazine in March 1845, the editor in July, and in October the owner. At year's end the magazine died for lack of capital. Poe's only chance to own and run a periodical was over, and he felt exhausted and depressed. Virginia's illness was progressing; now she suffered night sweats and chills. Literary rivals satirized Poe in print as a vicious drunk; he sued one detractor for libel and won damages, but that helped his reputation little. A series of literary women befriended the Poes; some were generous helpers, but others, failing in flirtations with Edgar, turned vindictive. One sent malicious anonymous letters to the dying Virginia; others wrote poison-pen missives to Edgar's friends and colleagues for the rest of his life.

Edgar himself became so sick in 1846 that for most of the year he couldn't write, let alone hold a job. The winter was cold. A visitor found Virginia feverish on a straw bed, warmed only by Poe's old army coat and their tortoiseshell cat. The *Saturday Evening Post* appealed for help for the Poes, saying Edgar was "dangerously ill with brain fever" and Virginia in the last stage of consumption. They asked the public to ignore tales of Poe being a drunkard. They had seen that even one glass of wine made him instantly excited, almost demented; he had no control over this and later remembered little or nothing. Normally he was quiet, considerate, gentlemanly, and "perfectly self-possessed in all other respects." Some people donated cash and a blanket, but by early 1847, Virginia was past help. At the end, she made her mother promise to care for Edgar; she told him that he must go on living, and that he would need another woman's love to do so.

When she died on January 30, Poe collapsed utterly. He couldn't bear being alone, and Mrs. Clemm and a family friend named Louise Shew would sit by his bed till he fell asleep. If they didn't watch him, he wandered off to weep hysterically at Virginia's grave. The "brain fever" he had suffered for a year became worse than ever. Mrs. Shew, who had some nursing experience, noticed that when his pulse stopped racing, it became irregular. She reported this to a doctor at New York University medical school, and he confirmed her suspicion that Poe had a brain lesion, which explained why he responded to sedatives or stimulants "with insanity." The fever, she claimed, resulted from the cold and hunger he had endured trying to provide for Virginia.

As in past adversities, Poe drew on immense reserves of energy and resiliance. By spring he seemed healthier and was scrabbling for survival money again, trying to start a magazine, and writing his prose poem "Eureka." He finished the work, for which he received fourteen dollars and mixed reviews, and plowed on at writing and lecturing. But often he suffered agonies of emptiness and grief. In June he wrote to Mrs. Shew that "unless some true and tender, and pure womanly love saves me, I shall hardly last a year longer alive!" He did not find another "angel to my forlorn and darkened nature," and would outlive Virginia by only two years, in a feverish quest for love and domestic security.

Traveling as a lecturer, Poe met many women eager to console a famous poet so elegant, sad, and needy. In Providence there was Sarah Helen Whitman, an attractive widow of forty-five who wrote verse and fainted promiscuously. They whipped up extravagant scenes in their self-consciously literary courtship. In a cemetery, Poe called her his second Helen, swore his love, and proposed. She hesitated, giving him time to cool, and in Lowell, Massachusetts, he developed a warmer, more geniune love for Mrs. Nancy ("Annie") Richmond. In November 1848, Poe begged Annie to leave her husband for him; otherwise, he said, he would have to keep his promise to marry

Mrs. Whitman. Annie was touched, but not about to run off with the increasingly frantic poet. She gently refused and made him promise to marry Mrs. Whitman; Poe made her promise in turn to come to him on his deathbed. She may have thought this mere rhetoric, but he was on the edge of a nearly fatal bout of physical and mental sickness.

Rejected by Annie, Poe spent a tortured night in a hotel room, bought two ounces of laudanum, and traveled by train to Boston. There he wrote to Annie, holding her to her promise, and swallowed half of the opiate, intending to take the rest if she failed to appear. But even half was a dose so massive that Poe threw it up in the street on the way to the post office, and he never mailed the letter. He arrived in Providence so sick that Mrs. Whitman set aside the defamatory letters she'd received from his old enemies and called a doctor. He diagnosed "cerebral congestion," and a neighbor cared for Poe as he recovered — with no memory, he wrote to Annie, of anything since taking the laudanum, but knowing "I am so *ill* — so terribly, hopelessly ILL in body and mind."

But again Poe apparently recovered physical and mental health. Mrs. Whitman said she would marry him if he swore off alcohol, and he agreed. But as soon as he was back at Fordham, he wrote to "my *pure, virtuous, beautiful, beautiful sister* Annie," begging her to come to him. Secretly Mrs. Clemm wrote to her as well, asking that she write Poe often, for he had returned home terribly changed. Annie remained Poe's confidante, but nothing more, and in December he returned to Providence reluctantly. Mrs. Whitman's family insisted that he renounce any claim to her property and sign a temperance pledge. He did both, but the next day, perhaps in defiance of their humiliating treatment, drank a glass of wine. Someone tipped off the Whitmans, there was a melodramatic scene of mutual accusations, and the engagement was off. By Christmas Poe was back at Fordham, swearing in a letter to Annie to "shun the pestilential society of *literary* women."

During the first six months of 1849, Poe worked productively, creating "For Annie" and "Annabel Lee," but still in beggarly straits. America's best poet and critic agreed to write a second series of *Marginalia* for two dollars a page; the work was printed, and he was never paid. Late in June, Poe left for Richmond, seeking lecture fees and magazine backers, but another physical and mental nightmare gripped him. A few days later he turned up haggard at the office of editor John Sartain in hot, cholera-stricken Philadelphia. He begged Sartain to cut off his mustache and hide him from two men who meant to kill him. Poe confided that he had been in Moyamensing prison, where a radiant young woman spoke to him in a dream from a stone tower. Soon he was sufficiently recovered to tell Sartain the whole thing had been a delusion (and indeed there is no record of his having been in Moyamensing). But on July 9 he wrote to Mrs. Clemm:

> My *dear, dear* Mother — I have been *so* ill — have had the cholera, or spasms quite as bad, and can now hardly hold the pen. . . .
>
> I was never really *insane,* except on occasions where my heart was touched.
>
> I have been taken to prison once since I came here for getting drunk; but *then* I was not. It was about Virginia.

On July 14 he arrived in Richmond, still wretchedly sick, and sent Mrs. Clemm one of the two dollars remaining from ten Srtain had given him. On July 19, finally recovering, he wrote to her, "For more than ten days I was totally deranged although I was not drinking one drop

. . . all was hallucination, arising from an attack which I had never before experienced." No one is sure what happened to Poe in those weeks, but obviously he suffered severe physical sickness and an episode of full-blown psychosis.

By late July, a fitter Poe was setting up lectures and being lionized in his home town. He also joined a temperance society and resisted marination in local hospitality with only a few lapses. In September he met Elvira Royster, the love of his teens, now the widow Elvira Shelton. Though still dreaming of Annie, he courted Elvira with his usual romantic worship, and they became engaged. He wrote rhapsodically to Mrs. Clemm that he, she, and Elvira would all live together — somewhere near Annie! During the past year, he had increasingly taken this hectic, disoriented tone. Still, it remained intermittent, and many people described him as healthy, self-possessed, and charming. And as always, he could rise from disaster with boyish confidence: "Although I feel ill, and am ground into the very dust with poverty, there is a sweet *hope* in the bottom of my soul."

But he was also often at the mercy of inner desperation and chaos, and preoccupied with death. He gave a successful lecture on September 24 but seemed nervous and pale. The next day, he told a friend that Rufus Griswold, his successor years ago at *Graham's Magazine,* had agreed to be his literary executor. The next night he was depressed and running a high fever; Elvira got him to postpone a trip to New York. When she came to visit him in the morning, she found he had already left on a boat for Baltimore. He was bound for his last nightmare.

Six days later, on October 3, there were congressional elections. A compositor for the *Baltimore Sun,* passing a polling place at a tavern, recognized Poe lying semiconscious in the street, wearing a cheap suit not his own. It has been guessed that Poe was a victim of "cooping," the wardheeler's trick of drugging or intoxicating men and dragging them from poll to poll, to vote at each. There is no evidence that Poe was drunk or drugged, but he was certainly very sick, and that day he was hospitalized. The next morning, according to an attending doctor, Poe passed from unconsciousness to delirium, sweating profusely and talking to "spectral and imaginary objects." Then he slept, and later entered a delirium so violent that two nurses had to hold him down. Early in the morning of October 7, the enfeebled Poe said only, "Lord help my poor soul," and soon after died. Two days later, he was buried in Baltimore. His grave went without a tombstone for a quarter century, and when one was finally erected, Walt Whitman was the only writer at the ceremony.

Poe had been much maligned in life, but that was mere prelude. His executor, the Reverend Rufus Griswold, launched a program of character assassination so fantastic that, as historian Perry Miller said, if there were no proof Griswold existed, we might think him one of Dickens's less plausible inventions. This abolitionist preacher turned editor and anthologist seems to have had no motive but a harsh review by Poe in 1843. The day of Poe's funeral, he wrote in the *New York Tribune* that Poe's death "will startle many, but few will be grieved by it." Poe, he said, had been a gifted writer, but his work, like his character, was gloomy and without humanity. He had been sickly, destitute, thin and pale "even to ghastliness," arrogant, gnawed by envy and ambition. Cynical, amoral, thinking himself damned, he walked the streets "in madness or melancholy, with lips moving in indistinct curses."

This article, widely reprinted, was just Griswold's first shot. In 1850, in Poe's collected works, he enlarged the portrait, quoting as evidence letters he had altered or completely invented. Compared to the sage, forbearing Griswold, Poe seemed irascible, fawning, and vain. His work was sensational and flawed, and he showed "scarcely any virtue in either his life or his writings." He had been expelled from his university for drinking and gambling; had deserted from the army; blackmailed a famous literary woman; plagiarized Longfellow; perhaps committed incest with his stepmother; died of a drunken debauch.

Longfellow protested the plagiarism charge, and Poe's friends and colleagues described him not only as a great artist but as gentle, industrious, and scrupulously courteous; though drinking affected him terribly, he had done it only sporadically. These replies drew little attention, while Griswold was quoted and believed everywhere — after all, Poe himself had appointed Griswold to his task. Griswold's lies and forgeries went undetected for a century, and even people who wanted to show Poe fairly repeated his libels.

Some writers didn't even aim at fairness, but at making Poe an example. A doctor who'd known Poe made him a cautionary case in temperance lectures. A much-quoted Scots cleric named Gilfillan called him a "swine" who "died as he had lived, a raving, cursing, self-condemned, conscious cross between the fiend and the genius." Then he charitably wished peace "even to the well-nigh putrid dust of Edgar A. Poe." Soon it was claimed that Poe had been a drug addict, neglected the dying Virginia, and committed incest with Mrs. Clemm. Until the 1940s, and sometimes beyond, he would be portrayed as a bizarre, heartless madman who died drunk in a gutter.

How did Poe become a twisted face on the barroom floor? It started with resentment of his harsh integrity as a critic and gossip of chronic alcoholism. It continued because America needed its first native example of the mad, wicked artist. With Romanticism, the artist became a mythic figure, a tortured rebel against social convention. Poe was the first major American writer who didn't live in apparent respectability, the first not to spout the virtues praised by Whittier and Emerson. To Victorian Gradgrinds who saw biography as a tool of moral persuasion, Poe was a threat to moral hygiene and a perfect example of artistic wrong and rot. As a critic said a few years after his death, he had "mercilessly exposed the depths and secrets of the heart . . . the black gulfs and chasms of our spiritual nature," instead of fulfilling art's true mission, "the promotion of joy and gladness." Baudelaire wasn't entirely wrong in calling Poe a martyr to a "barbarous realm equipped with gas fixtures." Unlike Baudelaire and Byron, Poe never wanted his reputation.

Abroad, Poe's success was grand and unequivocal. Tennyson called him the equal of Catullus and Heine; Hardy, Conrad, Dostoevski, Valéry, Mallarmé, and Mann admired him enormously. True, some of Poe's French admirers projected their own ideas onto him; Barbey d'Aurevilly called his work a flower that took on strange new colors because its roots had been dipped in poison. But Poe was not a diabolist, a Decadent, or even a Bohemian. He was just poor and unlucky. Like Chopin, he was an aristocrat as a man and artist, a formalist who made innovative masterpieces in miniature. Like Chopin, because he spun dizzying Romantic inventions over his meticulous structures, he was misperceived, even by admirers, as florid or disordered.

At home, Poe long remained a literary bad citizen. Twain, Whitman, and Mencken diluted their praise with demurrals. Bryant and Whittier called him cold, demoniacal.

Emerson dismissed him as "the jingle man," and Lowell lampooned him in his "Fable for Critics":

Here comes Poe with his Raven, like Barnaby Rudge,
Three-fifths of him genius, and two-fifths sheer fudge.

Henry James deemed enthusiasm for Poe the sign of "a decidedly primitive state of reflection," and T. S. Eliot called his achievement that of a "highly gifted person before puberty."

Some of the criticisms have a measure of truth, yet "The Raven" is the best-known American poem, and "To Helen" one of the best. Poe remains one of the great American poets, a shaper of the short story, the creator of detective fiction, a founder of science fiction, and his age's best critic and editor. Like Byron and Rousseau, he soared beyond his flaws to influence world literature. As the vitriol has been scraped off his portrait, his literary stock has risen. Now critics speak of his having anticipated modern science in "Eureka," pure poetry and Symbolism in his verse, surrealism and depth psychology in his tales, and the New Criticism in his essays. Shaw justly said that his verse sometimes alarms the reader by fainting with its own beauty, but he "produced magic where his greatest contemporaries produced only beauty," and that magic has seized every generation of readers, despite detractors and critics.

If history offers lessons, there is surely one in how views of Poe's life and work changed along with society and science. The earliest interpretations were more mythic than scientific. It was only about the time of Poe's birth that the first pioneers of psychiatry unfettered the insane, calling them ill rather than possessed by demons. The idea of possession lingered. Nathaniel Willis, one of Poe's first biographers, said he was "inhabited by both a devil and an angel." Other writers, mixing moral and psychological speculation, described him as a Dr. Jekyll under whose Hyde lay some insane source of eerie, morbid writings.

There had long been a protopsychology that linked personality to physique and body functions. Hippocrates and Empedocles said personality was determined by the four humors: blood, phlegm, yellow bile (choler), and black bile (dark choler); from this theory we retain the words sanguine, phlegmatic, choleric, and melancholic. The idea of constitutional character types remained popular into and beyond Poe's lifetime. Lowell reflected it when he said that in Poe "the heart somehow seems all squeezed out by the mind." This idea of an innately unbalanced character, ingenious yet heartless, would be repeated by many critics and biographers.

In Poe's time, the idea was finally being accepted that the brain, rather than other organs and their humors, was the seat of emotion and behavior. One of the first fruits of this idea was phrenology, developed by Franz Joseph Gall and Johann Spurzheim in Germany in the late eighteenth century. Though laughed at today, it was a half-step toward science, claiming that since each mental function was ruled by a specific part of the brain, the power of those functions showed in the contours of the skull. Phrenology was popular with many laymen and scientists, including Poe, who had his cranium interpreted at least once. A related theory, physiognomy, inferred the nature of the mind not through the skull but the face. Poe satirized physiognomy in a little essay about the alleged ancient Greek science of "Rinosophia," reading the character by the shape of the nose. Not everyone shared Poe's skepticism; Captain Fitzroy of the *Beagle* almost refused to take Darwin as ship's naturalist because his nose didn't show "sufficient energy and determination."

As late as 1906, a phrenological study of Poe was written by one Oliver Leigh, who claimed to see the artist-demon split in Poe's character in his asymmetrical face. The swollen left side of the forehead, he said, gave rise to the grotesque, unbalanced aspect of Poe's life and work; the square side housed Poe the builder. One portrait of Poe does show such asymmetry, but the perspective is primitive, and the rest of Poe looks equally out of kilter. A late daguerreotype shows an apparent bulge at Poe's right temple, with an indentation below it. Another picture shows the bulge on the left. A drawing from another daguerreotype suggests an odd bulge on both sides; a few decades ago, someone claimed this was the mark of a traumatic forceps delivery that damaged Poe's brain at birth.

Other pictures, however, show no asymmetries at all, and not one person who described Poe verbally mentioned odd bulges. The apparent deformations in some pictures may result from harsh lights and shadows on Poe's unevenly receding hairline. Yet Poe's great modern biographer, Arthur Quinn, read into one picture the alleged asymmetry on which Leigh based his book — one eye perhaps a bit bleary, the mouth and mustache maybe drooping on the same side. A droop on one side of the face might reflect neurological damage, but look as I may at that picture, I can be sure only of an unevenly trimmed mustache surrounded by inference.

Phrenology and physiognomy were dead ends, but nineteenth-century psychology had little more to offer. If the brain governed thought and feeling, mental illness must be caused by a brain lesion. Freud's professor of neurology confidently taught that all mental disease rose from abnormal circulation of blood to the brain. Still, there was no way to examine the living brain, so the study of the mind remained a castle of diagnostic categories. It could give little help to biographers, let alone clinicians. And then, as always, the spirit of the time pervaded science; even theories of brain function remained as much moral as clinical.

The Western equation of sanity and reason couldn't explain the person who was rational, even brilliant, yet disturbed in feelings or behavior — the otherwise "sane" alcoholic, kleptomaniac, or sexual nonconformist. In 1835, English psychologist J. C. Pritchard invented the concept of moral insanity, a "morbid perversion of natural feelings" without loss of reason. In our century, the words psychopath and sociopath would be used similarly, drawing on moral and social standards as much as medical ones. The term moral insanity seemed to fit the Poe depicted by Griswold and his heirs, and that was the diagnosis in the first psychiatric study of Poe, by the dean of British psychiatry, Dr. Henry Maudsley.

Maudsley's essay appeared in 1860 in the *American Journal of Insanity* (the word psychiatry was relatively new and uncommon). Maudsley thought that mental ills arose from diseases or toxins that affected the nervous system. He also held the common view, later reinforced by pioneer research in genetics, that heredity caused insanity — or at least a predisposition to it (neurasthenia) that might be brought out by alcohol, drugs, exhaustion, sexual "excess," or other real or imagined strain on the brain. Into the 1920s, psychiatrists would routinely repeat Maudsley's opinion that Poe was a case of innate neurosis whose "bad heredity" led to alcoholism that further damaged the brain.

There were other, more lurid theories of genetic affliction. In 1875 it was first suggested that Poe suffered epilepsy, then thought a curse of genetic degeneration. A doctor who treated Poe in 1848 denied that he had the disease, but Poe's tales, like his drinking and psychotic episodes, would be called the result of epileptic hallucinations. Essayist James Huneker, who as a boy had known some of Poe's old friends in Philadelphia, said in print that masked epilepsy accounted for Poe's problems, but in a letter confided that he thought the real problem was syphilis. Occasional gossip about epilepsy and syphilis continued sporadically. Considering the straw man Poe had become for moralists, it's surprising there wasn't more.

Early in this century, Poe's first exhaustive biographers repeated the already widespread idea that he had been a drug addict — again, because of a genetic taint. In 1925, in a book called *Genius and Disaster: Studies in Drugs and Genius,* Jeanette Marks said Poe's life showed the impact of drugs on a brain lesion, and "Every paragraph of 'The Fall of the House of Usher' writes itself down as a drug work." Actually, only a few unreliable witnesses to Poe's life claimed he ever took opiates, though they were as easily obtained in his day as aspirin is now. Even Thomas Dunne, a physician who knew Poe, hated him, and publicly attacked his morals and sanity, called the drug charge a "baseless slander." Poe's ignorance of how much laudanum to take without throwing it up hardly seems the act of an addict.

Debate persists about genetic predisposition to some physical and mental ills, but evidence now leans heavily against the simple, direct inheritance of epilepsy and psychosis. One of the worst pressures on Poe may have been his own lifelong fear of bearing a hereditary flaw; in his day, belief in inherited traits and ills was powerful, and he shared it with his biographers. His mother had died of tuberculosis, then thought hereditary and somehow shameful. His father and brother were probably heavy drinkers; one of Poe's cousins wrote that alcohol was the family's curse. Poe's sister was mildly retarded, never developing mentally much beyond age twelve. Poe's sense of doom may have been partly a gnawing anxiety that he was fated to suffer consumption, drunkenness, imbecility, or madness.

By the late nineteenth century, the ideas of moral insanity and genetic neurasthenia had done what little they could to explain illness and behavior. A revolution came when psychoanalysis offered theories not of fixed traits but of emotional dynamics and personality development. It is difficult now to imagine the initial shock; today even many who say they reject analysis take for granted such analytic concepts as the unconscious, repression, compensation, paranoid projection, and childhood sexuality.

Analysis became popular in the twenties, as an anti-Victorian rebellion looked hopefully behind every appearance for the erotic, aberrant, and antisocial. Many people wanted to believe, as Freud had asserted, that civilization exists at the cost of impulse, and that dark, primitive cravings skulk behind the noblest facade. Yet even as twenties iconoclasts attacked their parents' moralism, they were sometimes just as judgmental and doctrinaire. Many analytic works on Poe resemble those of Victorian clerics, with adjustment usurping the throne of God, and neurosis the lair of the devil. When analytic ideas were misused, Poe, with his usual luck, took a posthumous pounding.

Freud published his trailblazing study of da Vinci in 1910, and two years later the journal *Imago* appeared, containing studies of artists as if they were patients, their art as if it were fantasy or dream. By the early forties, there had been a half-dozen analytic books and many more

articles on Poe — still, of course, Poe as depicted by Griswold. The most scholarly effort was by Freud's French
disciple Marie Bonaparte. Treating Poe and his narrators
as if they were one, she confidently claimed that his life
had been shaped by love for his dying mother, and that
he had been an impotent "sado-necrophile." Relentlessly,
mechanically, she applied Freudian templates to Poe's work
and decided that he often wrote about sea voyages because
he had a mother fixation, and the sea is a mother symbol.

Amateur analysts had a field day. The most widely read
was critic Joseph Wood Krutch, who sounded less like a
clinician than a hanging judge. His Poe, in a book subtitled
A Study in Genius, was a walking disease, painted with
venomous contempt. It made Poe's father a degenerate,
his sister an imbecile, Virginia a sexless little dope with a
"pale, unhealthy face" who "babbled pleasantly with the
childishness of arrested development." The poet's problems had begun with childhood humiliations and were
aggravated by impotence, which he hid by marrying someone first too young for sex and then too sick. When she
died, his "malformed soul" tumbled into drunken mis-
anthropy and "disgustingly weak dependence" on women.
Delusions overwhelmed him as he ceased to project his
madness in art, and it swamped his life.

There is something truly vengeful in Krutch's marathon
of belittlement. For instance, he claimed that Poe lacked
true learning and plagiarized in "ecstasies of mendacity."
Page after page contains such phrases as "psychopathic
case . . . shabby outcast . . . diseased soul." This is the
meanest work in its genre, but not the silliest. Critic Leslie
Fiedler called "Annabel Lee" an example of "child-love,
necrophilia, and incest." A more benign psychoanalytic
theory held that the key to Poe was a hidden, frustrated
urge to be an actor, like his parents.

From several decades of analytic and pseudoanalytic writings emerged a sad picture of Poe, fragments of which are still repeated ad libitum in literary criticism. When not quite three, Poe was traumatized by seeing his mother vomit blood, die, and be carried off by men in black. His upbringing left his vanity scarred, his ambition swollen. A sadist and misfit, he hid his insanity in his art. Impotent, he hid his inadequacy in the skirts of a child-wife and a substitute mother. Finally he became as mad as his maddest narrators.

Even in the twenties, some people objected. Edmund Wilson questioned Krutch's tendency to reduce genius to a bag of quivering kinks and failings. Such writers' savage reductionism does leave one wondering whether they were uncovering Poe's fantasies or indulging their own. Freud himself had warned, in his preface to Bonaparte's book, that analysis could not explain the mystery of genius, only why it chose certain themes. Despite the warning, most of the analytic writers violated both psychoanalysis and art.

They violated analysis by claiming to draw from books what must be learned directly through hundreds of hours with a living patient. They violated art by failing to see that as a book is not a patient, its contents are not dreams or projective tests. An artist transforms his life and imagination in a process that baffles science and artists alike. Although it is tempting to equate art and artist, no one suggests that Joyce was a transsexual because he created Molly Bloom, or Faulkner an impotent rapist because he wrote *Sanctuary*. Yet people freely assumed that Poe was Roderick Usher. Back in 1850, critic C. Chauncey Burr wrote, "I perceive not why the competent critic should fall into this error. Of all authors, ancient or modern, Poe has given us the least of himself in his works. He *writes* as an *artist.*" Truly, Poe's works were anything but personal outpourings; he did not even use a fictional persona, as Twain and Whitman did. He was a self-conscious artificer and constant reviser, bent on creating effects in the reader.

Some bits of the Poe scenario inferred by analysts are plausible, but are they true? We don't know that Poe saw his mother vomit blood and die. There is no evidence that he was impotent. We have plentiful testimony that he was sane, brilliant, and productive most of his life. He wrote with genius in a great variety of forms and tones, which no psychotic can do. This has not squashed wild analytic speculations. Art does reveal something about an artist, but in a partial and refractive way; it is as much a mask as a confession.

Behind much psychologizing of Poe lurked the belief that genius and madness are allied. The idea goes back at least to ancient Greece, and nineteenth-century Romantics cultivated the vision of a demonic creator whose gift rose from a dungheap of illness. It has comforted the mediocre and envious, who sourly like to think that great gifts are balanced out by great failings. But the "fine madness" of creation is not the anguish and disorder of the psychotic. Creative people in all fields keep an ability to tap the preconscious, magical part of the mind, which so many others shut away as childlike and threatening. The West has always feared the loss of conscious controls, though madness is more often a disorder of the emotions than of logic. Many of us briefly regain touch with the preconscious at times of strong emotion; in that sense, as Shakespeare said, the lunatic, lover, and poet "are of imagination all compact." But the artist doesn't create only when distraught or in love, and he has enormous powers of concentration and organization.

For every Van Gogh or Nietzsche, who became truly mad, there is a T. S. Eliot or J. S. Bach, with the habits of a banker. A century of studies of geniuses in fields from poetry to mathematics have shown that as a group they are as fit and sane as other people. Despite the myth that great artists are, in Thomas Mann's words, great invalids, art is not a symptom but a triumph and fulfillment. Poe agreed with Dryden's idea that "Great wit to madness nearly is allied," but considered wit, or isolated talent, mere "pseudo-genius." True genius, he said, is eminently sane and balanced.

Analytic excesses in studying Poe were finally answered by a change in the practice of biography. Through most of history, biographies were deliberately didactic. The idea that they should, like history, use the methods and standards of scientific research rose chiefly from nineteenth-century German scholarship and had flowered in American universities by the 1940s. Detection and documentation took the place of moralizing and metaphysics. What biography lost in thematic grandeur, it gained in accuracy. A model of such work was the life of Poe by Arthur Hobson Quinn of the University of Pennsylvania. When it appeared in 1941, Quinn was a distinguished elder of literary scholarship, and this volume of almost 800 pages, his last major work, began a new era in the study of Poe.

If it could be checked, Quinn hunted it down. He found maps of old Richmond to learn just where Elizabeth Poe died; sought letters and memoirs from collateral descendants of Poe and his friends; examined the originals of letters routinely reprinted from book to book. He even sent "Eureka" to such eminent scientists as Sir Arthur Eddington to test the common American literary judgment that it was half-mad pseudoscience.

Biographies such as Quinn's are often accused of scanting larger truths for the sake of laundry-list precision. This is sometimes true, but well-researched books have no corner on mediocrity, and one cannot build wisdom on a ground of error. Quinn had the good fortune that often finds a scrupulous scholar: new facts produced new truth and left previous works obsolete.

Quinn's most dramatic discovery was Griswold's forgeries; he also proved some other damaging accounts of Poe to be spiteful gossip. He reported an expert consensus that "Eureka" revealed high scientific learning and was in some ways ahead of its era's conventional thinking. But most important was Quinn's cumulative sifting of massive evidence on Poe's work, loves, health, and drinking. As if he had turned a kaleidoscope, the facts formed a new pattern. Quinn's Poe was a vigorous prankster of a youth who went on to distinguish himself at everything he tried except making money — as a poet, journalist, editor, even as a soldier. Finally he was eroded by terrible trials that would have soon broken most men, yet he kept many of his gifts and strengths to the end. Despite some warts, he appeared touchingly courageous and warm. He could also be thin-skinned and vindictive, which Longfellow attributed to "the irritation of a sensitive nature, chafed by some indefinite sense of wrong." But the wrongs were quite definite, and few of Poe's critics ever had to endure anything like them.

Plagued by personal vendettas, poverty, and sickness, Poe overproduced for people who misprized or envied his gifts. Editor George Graham wrote in retrospect that because Poe couldn't be a toady and a hack, he ended his life with a justified sense of having been ill-used and put aside by lesser men. Graham owed Poe such testimony.

When Virginia had her first hemorrhage, Poe asked him for an advance on his salary, and Graham, according to Poe, "not only flatly but discourteously refused."

It would have been strange if death and melancholy hadn't tinged Poe's life and work. He lost his parents, stepparents, brother, Mrs. Stannard, Elvira, Virginia, and Annie. Even without analytic concepts, it is easy to understand that he desperately craved a home, family, and transcendent devotion that blended lover and soul-mate. But these were not fantasies that turned away from life. He found real love and haven with Virginia. She was a child when they met, but by her middle teens had become remarkably lovely and mature — dark-haired, dark-eyed, affectionate, and charming. She was no simpleton; Edgar had taught her French, Italian, and mathematics, and she sang, played the piano, and wrote intricate amateur verse. According to frequent visitors to their home, she and Edgar were passionately in love. That she was younger and a cousin brought no cries of child-seduction or incest during the Poes' lives, and marriages between cousins and by girls in their early and middle teens are not rare today.

We know nothing of Edgar's and Virginia's sex lives. Poe was prim but intensely romantic in a way typical of his times; his ecstatic idealizing is like that of Keats, Longfellow, and countless other Romantic poets. Allen Tate has also suggested that it reflected the traditional Southern ideal of the pure woman. Quinn believed that if any of Poe's writings describes him and Virginia, it is the story "Eleonora," with its ring of clearly sexual passion. Those who say Poe had a Lolita complex ignore his love for women his age and older; those who say he sought mothers ignore Virginia and Elvira. What Poe did ravenously crave was love, and he kept losing it. That had something to do with his drinking.

Poe's first problem with drinking occurred in 1835, when deeply depressed because he might lose Virginia. By 1843, occasional binges were harming his personal and professional life; he was now riding the ghastly seesaw of Virginia's remissions and relapses. He wrote in a letter in 1848:

> Each time [Virginia relapsed] I felt all the agonies of her death — and at each accession of the disorder I loved her more dearly & clung to her with more desperate pertinacity. But I am constitutionally sensitive — nervous in a very unusual degree. I became insane, with long intervals of horrible sanity. During those fits of absolute unconsciousness, I drank, God only knows how often or how much. As a matter of course, my enemies referred the insanity to the drink rather than the drink to the insanity.

Like many writers, Poe dramatized his life, to the confusion of biographers. His letters and his friends' recollections show that he was far from insane during most of Virginia's sickness, but his sensitive psyche was tormented by grief and hardship, and this led to sporadic but more frequent drinking. Recall his extraordinary sensitivity to alcohol. Many have called Virginia's death a trauma that dissolved his life into psychosis and alcohol abuse, but Quinn proved that both problems remained episodic even during his last two years.

I think that Quinn gave too little weight to Poe's long, severe "brain fever" during Virginia's last year, which finally brought a diagnosis of "brain lesion." Only after that did Poe have bouts of psychosis, always associated with physical illness but not always, to our knowledge, with alcohol. I have asked many doctors to attempt a modern diagnosis but none felt they had enough evidence even to try. Poe may well have suffered meningitis, a brain tumor, or any of a dozen other neurological ills that progressively undermined his physical and mental well-being. Whatever the disease, it was probably largely responsible for his final ordeals.

In the decades since Quinn, studies of Poe have given increasing weight to social history, attributing less to Poe's psyche and more to his times. Ellen Glasgow said long ago that Poe, in his formalism, sentimentality, aloofness, and intensity, belonged to his epoch and especially to the South. His Southern upbringing also hobbled his career. During the growing sectionalism that led to the Civil War, Poe was the first major Southern writer to go North, where none of the dominant New England writers save Lowell made a generous place for him. This may have contributed to his lifelong feeling of being uprooted and an outsider. Poe never fully belonged anywhere. He was the orphan of actors, who were third-class citizens; an American boy in England; an English-bred boy in Virginia; never adopted; raised in a class he didn't belong to; an aristocrat cast into pauperdom, working in a profession then thought one cut above entertainers; a dark, revolutionary Romantic in the day of Whittier and Emerson.

Many scholars now deny Poe's identity with his characters and stress how his fiction reflected the era of Camille and of Frankenstein's monster. Even Van Wyck Brooks, who called Poe an example of bad heredity and maybe even a bad gestation, admitted that in Poe's time a young girl dying of consumption wasn't only a common literary theme but a common reality. Mario Praz, in *The Romantic Agony,* listed and analyzed the common themes of that period: monsters, vampirism, and terror; ancient families falling to ruin in their ancestral homes; a cultivated, fatal melancholy; passion between cousins and siblings; the entwining of love and death; fascination with decay, sado-masochism, and monomania; cruelty and amorality for their own sake. If Poe was mad because of his subjects, so were half of his greatest contemporaries.

Actually, Poe disliked Gothic excess; he even objected to Goethe's *Werther* as morbid. He began to make money by writing parodies of the grotesque fiction associated with such Germans as E. T. W. Hoffmann — in which, incidentally, first-person narrative was a common device. The tale "Berenice," Poe said, was "half banter, half satire." He may have written it not, as critics and analysts once claimed, because he had fantasies of pulling dead girls' teeth, but because he had read of just such a bizarre case in a Baltimore newspaper, and there was a fad for such tales. Scholars have now found sources for many of Poe's stories in news items and books of his time.

When Poe's stories appeared in a volume, he objected in the preface to being criticized for "Germanism" and gloom: "I maintain that terror is not of Germany, but of the soul." This was probably a half-truth meant to legitimize his sort of fiction and assert his originality. He had begun with mixed intentions, to spoof horror tales yet use their most effective elements (something now common in sophisticated suspense films, which blend terror and touches of self-parody). But Poe's gift for creating moods with convincing detail took him beyond satire. Like many other writers, he found that tales of terror and fantasy could portray dreamlike states, from the hellish to the paradisiacal.

Many European writers were doing the same thing, but few Americans. Poe's tales of obsession, ecstasy, and the "imp of the perverse" struck sparks in Baudelaire and Dostoevski. Predictably, they were less winning to admirers of Julia Ward Howe, as were his attempts to produce in verse a music that was unearthly, pure, and sad. True, Poe might have written about other things, even for money, and there were grief and horror enough in his life and imagination. Still, he was the first American example of a mood that swept through Western art, and it is as much a matter of cultural history as of individual psychology.

Today that seems reasonable, but many views that now look biased or silly once seemed enlightened. If our present picture of Poe ever seems stunningly wrong-headed, it will probably be because of something we consider self-evident. It may even be our tendency to normalize Poe. In recent decades, history, psychology, and social science have had an orgy of relativism, of empathy for people and cultures unlike the mainstream of our own society. Some have tried to normalize the emotional, sexual, and social deviant with muscular moralism. Precisely because I can't believe we are wrong in rehabilitating Poe, I try to keep some reserve of doubt.

Yet I have found evidence that bolsters my view of Poe, showing that he could indeed have suffered a problem many doubt even exists — a constitutional inability to handle alcohol that made him seem drunk and sick even if he drank lightly and occasionally (let alone, under stress, heavily or regularly). In the early seventies, researchers began to study the one enzyme, alcohol dehydrogenase, that breaks down alcohol in the body, and how it is genetically controlled. The results brought to light a genetic state called alcohol dehydrogenase deficiency.

Researchers found three variations of the gene that determines alcohol breakdown, each most common in a different racial group. Most Caucasians have a gene that allows the body to handle high levels of alcohol. Many blacks have one that allows for a somewhat lower level (the evidence here is sketchier). Mongoloids have a gene that permits little alcohol in the body without severe symptoms from flushing to palpitations to dizziness — that is, becoming sick drunk. This should be no surprise, since such differences in reactions to other drugs have been found.

These variations explain what have often been called cultural variations in the use of alcohol. It was Caucasians who developed distilled spirits; their bodies can tolerate a high dose of alcohol. Orientals and Amerindians show the same symptoms after a drink of beer or wine as most Caucasians after a shot of liquor; there is considerable Asian folklore to this effect. It is the same low susceptibility to alcohol that causes many Indians' notorious reaction to liquor. Researchers have tested for cultural conditioning by giving alcohol tests to newborns of many racial and cultural backgrounds; the genetic force showed at birth.

As in so many genetic characteristics, the three racial populations are not uniform. In rough numbers, 15 percent of Mongoloids can tolerate higher levels of alcohol. About 5 percent of Caucasians have the same low threshold as Asians and Indians; if they follow normal Western drinking habits, they will react like Indians drunk on a taste of whiskey — and like Edgar Allan Poe.

The alcohol dehydrogenase deficiency syndrome still isn't widely known even among alcoholism researchers. Its relationship with alcohol abuse is yet unknown. However, the initial evidence is strong, and anyone who reads the scientific papers and knows Poe's life will have a flash of recognition. As we saw in studies of Goya, that flash doesn't guarantee accuracy. But I propose this syndrome as the best possible explanation of Poe's abnormal reaction to alcohol, and its crucial role in his life. When we put the syndrome in the context of a hard-drinking society and the apparent brain disease of Poe's last years, the fit is even better. Physical medicine may never identify with certainty Poe's late illness or his odd relationship with alcohol, but if further research strengthens my theory, it will help distinguish Poe the man from Poe the medical misfortune.

The future will judge, when better studies of Poe arrive. I hope even Quinn's excellent biography will be surpassed by one including what he scanted as beyond his competence — the thorough biohistory of Poe. It will draw on some approaches that were misused in the past, such as genetics and psychoanalysis. Genetics has come a long way since the nickel-in-a-slot simplicities of early inheritance theory. There is still argument between reductionist zealots and researchers who fully confront the complexities of behavior genetics. Personality and behavior do have some basis in the body — not in skull contours or simple genetic pedigree, but the interplay of genes, enzymes, hormones, nervous system, and environment.

Most psychoanalytic studies of Poe were dismally bad, but psychodynamic concepts are helpful if used cautiously and with understanding of the biographical facts and historical context. Doctrinaire classical analysis like Marie Bonaparte's is now rare. Eriksonian psychobiography has become popular; it has some of the same pitfalls but puts useful emphasis on identity formation and personality development. Ideally we will some day see a richly eclectic approach that draws on the best of Freud, neo-Freudianism, Adler, Sullivan, Erikson, and others, without scanting the medical and physical aspects of behavior and personality.

The ideal biohistory of Poe, then, will be wide-ranging

and balanced, giving a global sense of Poe's physical and mental life, his work, and his times. It will take nothing entirely for granted, including its strongest convictions. This book will be worth writing for two reasons. First, because such a study of anyone will be a model for biographers and set a new standard for readers. Second, because for a long time to come, if people are asked to name the first poet whose work they knew and loved, a vast number will still say Edgar Allan Poe, and they will want to know who he really was.

4

Mummy Powder, Mummy Blood

TOWARD A BIOHISTORY OF PEOPLES

DURING the past decade, the mummies of two ordinary Egyptians entered history after groups of scientists autopsied them thoroughly and ingeniously. Neither was a pharaoh, noble, or priest. One was a poor teenage weaver named Nakht who died 3,200 years ago. We don't even know the other's name, age, or occupation; he goes by the acronym PUM because the University of Pennsylvania's University Museum provided him for research. As individuals, Nakht and PUM don't matter to history; neither does their physical state in life or death. Nor were they the first mummies subjected to X-ray and scalpel; paleopathology, the study of people's health and habits through their physical remains, began a century ago. Nakht and PUM are memorable because the complex and imaginative team research on them suggests new ways to learn about entire vanished peoples.

However great the contribution to history and to other Large Matters, the study of mummies needs no justification. They hold a unique and universal fascination. In my childhood, I went often to the dimly lit mummy room of Philadelphia's University Museum to gaze at an eerie, wizened form with teeth and bits of skull peeking through the wrappings and blackened resins. Though frightening at first, it also evoked mystery and awe; this had once been a feeling, dreaming person like myself. Our society tries to hide death, especially from children; yet I, like every child, could recall the numb terror of first grasping that when I died, the world would die, for I wouldn't be here to see it. That mummy made me dwell in some oddly bearable way on life, death, and time beyond death.

Perhaps such experience with mummies underlies the theory that thoughts of immortality led to preserving the dead. I suspect that something less abstract made men overcome their reluctance to disturb the flesh of the dead and mummify their kings and priests, parents and children. Another theory holds that discovering naturally mummified bodies led to deliberate preservation. I imagine some aborigine who gazed for the first time at a natural mummy, not prepared, as I was, by pictures and history lessons. He probably screamed, fled, and prayed, in that order. Then, like me, he returned to look, and look again, losing fear, gaining awe and wonder, reflecting on the same things as I before that shrunken gesture of triumph over death and time. But this theory, too, has weak spots. Even the best of mummies is uninviting; I can't imagine it would rouse envy and emulation. Furthermore, mummification has been practiced in climates where natural preservation is rare or impossible.

Normally, nature abhors a mummy; it requires organic decay, lest the world vanish under mountains of dead plants and animals. Decomposition depends on bacteria, warmth, moisture, and chemical changes; sometimes extremes of dryness, cold, and heat interfere, and the result is a natural mummy. People and animals have been found frozen and virtually unchanged after centuries, even mil-

lennia, in polar ice. Natural mummies are most common
in the deserts of Egypt and the sands and mountains of
Peru. In temperate climates, the cool dryness of caves and
crypts has accidentally embalmed the dead; there are many
such natural mummies in Vienna and Kiev, and thousands
in catacombs beneath Palermo. The cathedral of Venzone,
in northern Italy, holds the natural mummies of some two
dozen people originally buried in vaults beneath the church
floor as long as six centuries ago.

Venzone may owe its mummies not only to cool crypts
but to the dehydrating action of a local fungus. Often
something in the environment thus helps embalm the dead.
Indians found in caves in Wyoming and Kentucky may
have been mummified by niter, sodium salts, and other
compounds in the soil. One of the most famous natural
mummies is the "Copper Man" discovered in 1905 in the
Chilean Andes. This miner died in a cave-in four hundred
years ago and lay where he fell, with his tools beside him;
the cave air and copper salts preserved him uncannily.
The world's most remarkably preserved bodies are those
dug up in northern Europe's peat bogs, where decaying
moss produces acids that kill bacteria and tan skin to a
fine leather. These Danes of the Iron Age, two thousand
years ago, seem only to sleep and could still be identified
individually by their fingerprints.

Perhaps in some places people did indeed realize that
dryness, heat, cold, cave burial, salt, certain minerals, and
alcohol all helped prevent decay, and applied these to their
dead, learning mummification by trial and error. It is significant that Egypt and Peru have the most artificial as
well as natural mummies. But on every continent, in places
dry and tropical, people have made mummies. A number
of societies in Melanesia and Australia traditionally dried
their chiefs in the sun and smoked them before fires, as

one cures game. In such climates, mummies lasted a few years at most; eventually the remains were buried or cremated, and the skull given to the nearest relative as a drinking cup full of fond memories. Here, I suspect, may lie the chief reason for making mummies. Many peoples have made a custom of keeping some piece of those they valued most, as relics to treasure or revere. It seems a logical step from the worldwide custom of saving ancestors' ashes or skulls to preserving their entire bodies. Perhaps concern for the afterlife was an afterthought, even a rationalization. When we lose those we love, we lose a part of ourselves; by keeping them, we conquer separation and loss.

Many peoples have made that attempt, in different ways and with different rationales. In northern China, two thousand years ago, a princess was sealed in a coffin containing a mercury solution; today her joints can be flexed, and the skin is so elastic that it rebounds from a finger's prodding. Until the turn of this century, some Japanese monks had themselves mummified so that they would be here to help the Buddha when he visits this world. The ancient Ainu, Aleuts, and Canary Islanders preserved their chiefs; the Scythians mummified their leaders along with concubines and dozens of retainers and horses. The Conquistadors saw mummified Inca kings displayed in Cuzco's main square and offered food, drink, and entertainment. And of course the Egyptians manifested their rulers' immortality by preserving their corpses. Those who think such behavior primitive should ponder the painstaking embalming (perhaps with paraffin) of Lenin and Eva Peron, whom mobs offer the same worship as that given to mummified saints in European churches.

I cannot leave this brief survey of mummies without mentioning a bizarre case that clearly served the wishes not of the living but the dead. Jeremy Bentham, the English philosopher who created Utilitarianism, willed that his body be dissected for the benefit of anatomy students, a gesture befitting his rabid rationalism. But he further directed that he be reduced to a skeleton and his head preserved entire, fitted with glass eyes, and remounted on the skeleton. This gruesome assemblage was to be dressed in Bentham's best clothes and brought out at every meeting of the Utilitarian Society. The utility of the request is obscure, but it was followed for more than a century after Bentham's death in 1832. The head was eventually replaced by a wax replica, for reasons utilitarian, esthetic, or merely hygienic.

In Bentham's day, doctors had learned how to interfere with decomposition, a skill the Egyptians had lost more than a thousand years earlier. How the Egyptians first learned remains a guess. The predynastic Egyptians buried their dead simply, in holes in the hot desert sand; they may have noticed that this often led to natural preservation. Around 3000 B.C., they began wrapping bodies in linen and placing them in coffins in subterranean burial chambers. There the bodies were not preserved as in the sand; perhaps that prompted efforts to embalm at least the divine pharaohs. Over two millennia, the Egyptians kept improving their methods, which eventually included removing the viscera and brain (which decay fastest), disinfecting the body by washing it in palm wine, dehydrating it in mineral salts, and sealing out moisture and air with wrappings, resins, and pitch. This took seventy days and much material and labor, so at first it was done only to pharaohs and high nobles and priests; eventually, faster and cheaper methods were devised for lesser citizens. It had become central to Egyptian belief that the soul was best served if the body endured in lifelike form. When mummification reached its height, packing was stuffed under the skin to compensate for shrinkage, and special care taken to preserve the appearance of the face, breasts, and genitals. A carefully painted mask might cover the face, perhaps as decoration, perhaps as a spiritual insurance policy against swathed anonymity.

All that art and labor eventually dwindled to a vague recollection. Around 1400 A.D., the Latin word *mummia* began appearing in English writings, meaning mummy powder. It came from an Arabic word for pitch; it has been suggested that pitch was used medicinally in classical times, and medieval doctors, perhaps thinking ancient pitch the best pitch, prescribed powder of pitch-embalmed Egyptians as a cure for everything from tuberculosis to bruises. By the late sixteenth century, Alexandrian merchants were busy digging up mummies and shipping them to apothecaries throughout Europe, where consumers had to beware of counterfeit *mummia* made from local cadavers.

By Shakespeare's time, the word mummy was being used for the preserved body itself. A century later, a few doctors in England and Germany began dissecting mummies to learn about Egyptian diseases and burial practices. The summa of this early research was the *History of Egyptian Mummies,* by Thomas Pettigrew, which appeared in 1834 with illustrations by the great Cruikshank. The medicinal use of *mummia* had ceased only recently; now European museums were acquiring mummies for display, though these were still seen primarily as curiosities, not sources of historical knowledge. To some, they were not even precious antiquities. In Canada, a rag shortage prompted manufacturers to use vast amounts of mummy wrapping in paper-making (we don't know the fate of the bodies), and mummies were even used as ships' ballast.

The modern study of mummies began in the late nineteenth century, after two great caches of royal mummies
had been discovered near Thebes. These were moved to
the Egyptian Museum in Cairo, where the British administration had recently founded a school of medicine. Several of the school's professors, especially anatomist Grafton
Elliot Smith and bacteriologist Marc Armand Ruffer, proceeded to lay the foundations of modern paleopathology.

Paleopathology was a new concept. Its pioneers had to
invent new methods, and to work without unwrapping the
magnificient royal mummies. One of their first hopes was
the recently discovered technique of X-ray pictures, or
radiographs. Egypt had only one X-ray machine, and one
night in 1904, Smith smuggled the rigid remains of Pharaoh Thutmosis IV into a cab and hustled it through the
dark streets to a nursing home, where he took the first,
hurried radiograph of a mummy. Ruffer invented a way
to rehydrate mummified tissue so that it could be studied
under the microscope, and his method is still used today.
Ruffer was also the first to discover parasites and bacteria
in mummy tissue. In 1910 he reported that he had found
in two nonroyal mummies the three-thousand-year-old eggs
of the schistosome that may have infected Napoleon during his Egyptian campaign.

Ruffer, Smith, and others discovered many interesting
facts, such as the presence of tuberculosis and perhaps
smallpox in ancient Egypt. These could enter medical history along with Napoleon's hemorrhoids, interesting and
perhaps significant, but hardly deepening one's view of
the past. Research on ancient Egypt's dead slackened after
the first few decades of pioneering work. The royal mummies weren't systematically X-rayed until the late 1960s,
when a new type of portable machine made the task prac-
tical. This was done not by Egyptologists or pathologists,

but by researchers from the University of Michigan School of Dentistry, who wanted to learn how human dentition has evolved. That turned out to be just one of many discoveries pointing to broad new possibilities in paleopathology.

This research rested on the fact that the conformation of the skull, facial bones, and teeth are stable hereditary traits, following racial and family patterns. Furthermore, the teeth retain a record of diet, nutrition, general health, and the environment's effects on the entire body — for instance, through telltale lines of arrested growth caused by disease or malnutrition. Michigan researchers, headed by James Harris and Kent Weeks, had been studying local schoolchildren to learn how their teeth revealed genetic and environmental influences. But Americans are genetically quite varied and offer few generations for study; Harris and Weeks needed groups with which to compare them. They had the good fortune to seek comparisons in Nubia, in what is now southern Egypt and northern Sudan.

In 1965, the building of the Aswan High Dam threatened to flood the temple of Abu Simbel; there were crash programs to salvage the area's archaeological remains, including five thousand skeletons and natural mummies that had been buried in the Nubian sands over a period of two thousand years. Nubia had long been a crossroads of northern Africa, with a complex but sketchily understood history linked to Egypt's. This intriguing place offered the Michigan researchers the remains of a hundred generations, and thus an opportunity to explore the evolution of a people and their changing patterns of physical health and disease. Harris and Weeks also arranged to study two thousand present-day Nubian children and won permission to X-ray the skeletons of the royal mummies in Cairo. They would then be able to compare ancient

Nubia's peasants to their rulers, the ancient Nubians to their descendants, and all of these to modern Americans. Studying the royal mummies offered still other avenues of research. Full-body X-rays can help reveal a person's age at death, sex, whether a woman has borne children, and signs of many diseases. The results might tell much about the pharaohs' health, racial origins, family relationships, and chronology.

The project demanded five seasons of painstaking labor in Egypt and many years of laboratory analysis in Ann Arbor by physical anthropologists, orthodontists, statisticians, and other specialists. The team took 149 measurements of each skeleton or mummy and many X-rays from a variety of angles, and they put the results through complex computer analysis. The results ranged from broad, important conclusions to fascinating trivia.

The researchers found that modern Nubians have smaller faces and jaws than their ancestors, and more crowded teeth. This confirmed the theory that everywhere the human jaw is becoming smaller, but the teeth are changing little, causing a predictable increase in certain dental problems. One might first think that this matters only to orthodontists and their stockbrokers. But dental configuration is a defining trait of each species, reflecting its adaptation to the environment. Changes in human dentition, which reflect diet and subsistence patterns, are as significant and revealing as changes in the human hand, brain, and sexual system.

The Nubian remains also showed that although many peoples had passed through their land, the Nubians had intermarried little and remained surprisingly homogeneous. Their dental problems did change, though, quite abruptly. Ancient Nubians had few caries, but they suffered from a condition rare in modern Americans. Because of coarse food and windblown sand that infiltrated their granaries and kitchens, their teeth wore down badly, sometimes almost to the gumline. This exposed the pulp and led to abscesses, chronic infection, and tooth loss; these conditions were so common and severe that they must have shortened many people's lives. Such wear still afflicts many Nubians, but they have a new problem as well. When children moved to new villages to escape Aswan's rising waters, their diets changed to include more sugar and refined food, and they began to develop the caries that have plagued Westerners for centuries. Thus the Nubian research confirmed that caries increase with a modern diet, but disproved that ancient peoples were necessarily better off with their natural diets.

Researchers expected to find very different health problems in ancient peasants and royalty, since the latter probably had richer diets and more sedentary lives. They were surprised to find that pharaohs and fellahin had the same dental woes; sand, knowing no class barriers, entered palace and hovel alike. Further surprises came from the search for clues to genetic and family relationships in the royal mummies' bones and teeth. Egypt's rulers did not, as scholars had long believed, represent one family tree. The nobles of the Old Kingdom (roughly 2680–2180 B.C.) were physically similar and probably related. Those of the New Kingdom (1600–1085 B.C.) are shown as looking alike in Egyptian paintings, but that was not the real case. Several dynastic lines show internal family resemblances in X-rays of their skulls and teeth, but as groups the dynasties were as physically varied as twentieth-century Americans.

Egyptian papyri had suggested that the royal family brought nobles from conquered nations to its court, and that some married into Egypt's ruling class. Now X-rays hinted where some of the genetic intruders came from.

Around 1600 B.C. Senakhtenre Tao, a commoner, won
Egypt's throne by driving the warlike Hyksos from Lower
Egypt and unifying the kingdom. His mummy has not been
found, but he and his wife Tetisheri started a line that
ruled for three centuries, and many of them, like Tetisheri
and her son Seqenenre Tao, had the characteristic protruding upper jaw and buck teeth of Nubia.

The Michigan team's X-rays confirmed some specific
historical points. For instance, Senakhtenre Tao's son was
throught to have died in battle. Radiographs revealed an
ax wound in his skull and a shattered cheekbone; there
were no signs of healing, so presumably he died of these
wounds or of others inflicted at the same time. But there
were also contradictions of presumed fact. Egyptologists
had thought that Thutmosis I ruled for a decade and died
at age fifty; according to X-rays, he died at eighteen. In
fact, X-rays disproved so many previous estimates of royal
longevity that the pharaohs' chronology, like their family
trees, demanded many revisions.

Some discoveries, though minor, remain tantalizing.
Normally, Egyptians above the lowest social class were
circumcised at puberty; but X-rays, which sometimes reveal soft tissues, showed that the pharaoh Ahmose was
uncircumcised. Perhaps Ahmose was not Egyptian by birth;
perhaps hemophilia or some other health problem prevented circumcision — X-rays also showed that he was
more delicately built than his father and his descendants.
A quite bizarre fact emerged from studying the mummies
of the priests of Amon, who around the eleventh century
B.C. became more powerful than the king. Historians had
believed that Makare, a woman variously described as a
high priestess or as a sister of a high priest, had died at
childbirth, and that the tiny mummy beside hers was the
infant. X-rays revealed the skeleton not of a baby but of

a female baboon. Harris and Weeks guess that the child lived and was raised secretly — perhaps it was illegitimate or a target of political intrigue — and the baboon was buried in its place.

In both Nubian and royal remains, Harris and Weeks found skeletal signs of spinal tuberculosis, mastoid infection, and perhaps gout, polio, and pituitary growth disorders. But they wanted to go beyond a mere list of diseases, combining X-rays, autopsy reports, and historical records to sketch out patterns of health, disease, and changing adaptation to the environment. They found that leprosy, rare or nonexistent in pre-Roman days, became relatively common in the post-Roman era. Schistosomiasis, which still plagues Egypt, was common in ancient peasants and royalty alike; the parasites probably entered children of all classes when they played in water. Pharaohs who reached early middle age weren't spared what we often think of as modern degenerative diseases. Many suffered advanced and painful arthritis. Blood-vessel disease was common, contrary to assumptions that it rises from urban stress and a modern high-fat diet. The Michigan team's study also allowed some comparisons with other ancient peoples. For instance, the Egyptians had many fewer leg fractures than such contemporaries as the early Anglo-Saxons; and when fractures did occur, healing without infection was far commoner in Egypt. Egyptian medical care was probably superior, but there may also have been fewer or less virulent germs in the environment.

Such discoveries began to offer a fuller picture of life and health in ancient Egypt. Still, science had not taken full advantage of the fact that a mummy is, as Harris and Weeks put it, a biological museum. The next major advance in paleopathology was an interdisciplinary group autopsy of a mummy. The project was less simple and less successful than researchers hoped, but it extended the Michigan team's efforts and spurred scientists around the world to form a loose partnership in reconstructing the health and history of ancient peoples.

The effort was sparked largely by the late Aidan Cockburn, a British-born scientist at Detroit's Wayne State University, who had been studying the evolution of infectious diseases. He and his wife Eve became interested in Egyptology, and in 1972 they enthusiastically announced that they and a few colleagues would autopsy a mummy at the University of Pennsylvania's University Museum.

Thousands of mummies had been autopsied between 1890 and 1920, but most in a cursory way, and without benefit of the ensuing explosion in medical knowledge. Still, carving this nameless mummy, dubbed PUM for the museum that donated him, attracted media attention and became a public event. The Cockburn team, unsure just how to proceed and what to look for, stumbled through their task hindered by television cameras and a class of visiting third-graders. They found a poorly preserved, eviscerated body and learned little except that they needed practice; this they gained in a second autopsy, without audience. Then in Detroit, in 1973, they worked on another mummy donated by the University Museum, which they called PUM II, and this time they learned a great deal.

Now the Cockburns worked with eleven other specialists, including a physical anthropologist, physiologist, pediatrician, and Egyptologist. Having X-rayed PUM II, they labored for seven hours with hammers, chisels, and a surgical saw to get through the resin that had been poured over the bandages and hardened like glass. They finally unwrapped a mummy in rather good condition, with the eyes and henna-painted nails intact. PUM II had been a man about five foot four who died when he was thirty-five or forty. Radioactive-carbon dating of his wrappings yielded a date of 170 B.C., which corresponded with the decorative style of his coffin. As in many mummies of that era, the viscera had been preserved in separate packages, and some tissues were preserved well enough for cell structure to be visible under a microscope.

Anyone who has dissected a cat or pig in a biology class knows how frustrating it can be to seek a nerve or a small organ even in a fresh cadaver. In a mummy, some tissues have dried and crumbled, others hardened like plastic, and all may be permeated by resin. There are also problems of contamination, ancient and recent, by fungi and bacteria, and of many kinds of pseudopathology. For instance, in X-rays taken before the unwrapping, PUM II's skull seemed to be fractured; the apparent fractures turned out to be mere scratches on the scalp, probably caused by the embalmers.

The cause of PUM II's death wasn't apparent, but he bore some obvious marks of illness. One was a perforated eardrum, then the earliest case on record; like many other ancient Egyptians, he must have suffered an acute ear infection some time in his life. The most interesting results came not from the initial autopsy but the many laboratory studies that followed. PUM II, like any modern patient, underwent tests, tests, tests. His body tissues were examined by some seventy-five scientists over five years.

First they studied the embalming materials. It turned out that the hardened outside substance, which had given off a sweet, pungent aroma when cut through by a saw, consisted chiefly of juniper resin, camphor oil, and myrrh. This sent researchers on a course of trying to reconstruct the native and imported woods, resins, and spices available in PUM II's time. Scientists could only puzzle over a small bundle of cotton that had been placed in the wrappings. Cotton was grown in India and South America long before PUM II's time, and was previously thought to have entered the Mediterranean world around the time of Christ. Perhaps the cotton was buried with PUM II precisely because it was rare and valuable. If it was grown in Egypt, the Mediterranean's agricultural and economic history will need revision. If it was imported, ancient Egypt had trade relationships previously unsuspected, perhaps with India.

Study moved from the outside of the mummy to the inside. PUM II's X-rays showed transverse lines in the bones of his thighs and shins. Such lines exist in virtually every human body and were first recognized a century ago. However, they were not studied intensively until the thirties, by H. A. Harris. These so-called Harris lines are actually scars left by interrupted growth. When a person is growing, each episode of illness or malnutrition stops bone growth; when health and growth resume, a line is left next to the growth cartilage at each end of the body's long bones. Paleopathologist Calvin Wells once likened an autopsy to a snapshot taken at the moment of death, and Harris lines to a motion picture of health and development from birth through adolescence. The correlation isn't perfect, but Harris lines in a person's bones do show roughly how many ills he suffered, and a line's distance from the end of the bone tells when it was laid down. PUM's bones had several Harris lines, but no more than most ancient Egyptians. By modern standards, they had a poor level of health and nutrition during childhood and the teens.

Paleopathologists moved from the X-rays to the bones themselves. They looked especially for signs of malaria, which has cruelly marked the history of the Mediterranean world. Chronic malaria causes anemia, which in turn may leave a telltale thickening of the skull's vault or a spongy pitting of the bones of the eye sockets. Both conditions have been found in many predynastic Egyptians and ancient Nubians. Their absence in PUM II doesn't mean that he never had malaria, but he probably wasn't enfeebled or killed by it, as were many of his contemporaries.

The search then went from PUM II's bones to his innards. It was no surprise to find signs of arteriosclerosis. Also unsurprising was the carbon in his lungs; fires for heating and cooking can create thick smoke in tents and huts, and carbon pollution is probably as old as the use of fire. It causes irritation but little permanent damage. But PUM II's lungs also showed, to researchers' surprise, the world's oldest case of silica damage. Today silicosis is still a potentially fatal disease of miners; since PUM II had uncallused hands, his lung disease probably wasn't occupational. The best explanation is that in his time, as today, Egyptians couldn't avoid inhaling sand from desert windstorms. Recently Israeli scientists have found silicosis in desert Bedouins, a condition they call Negev desert lung. Silicosis was later found in another Egyptian mummy, and future autopsies may show that the condition wasn't rare.

One package of viscera contained a piece of PUM II's intestine, which provided an interesting pathological clue, the egg of a parasitic roundworm, the first ever found in a mummy. Parasites usually decay along with their hosts, but the egg and cyst forms often survive better. The discovery of these forms can reveal not only health but diet and perhaps a person's socioeconomic standing. The study of another mummy, named ROM I, would later reveal a worm acquired from eating pork; the person had not been limited to the common Egyptian diet of milled cereal grains and occasional fish.

Next, the researchers studying PUM II became the first to study a mummy's tissues with a scanning electron microscope, which gives not only high magnification but a three-dimensional view. It allowed them to identify ancient bacteria and parasites, red and white blood cells, blood platelets, details of bone structure, and sometimes even the organelles within a cell. They searched PUM's liver tissue for virus particles, but with no success. This effort was related to another attempt at a technical first, a series of biochemical tests that might reveal ancient patterns of disease, diet, heredity, group migration or intermarriage, and adaptation to the environment.

The first step was to try to isolate proteins from PUM II's tissues, especially antibodies. The simplest and most effective antigen test was that for blood typing. Blood types, like dentition patterns, are stable genetic traits, and they exist in characteristic proportions in each genetic pool. Therefore blood-type profiles of a population over long periods may show whether they mingled with other peoples and whether a modern population in the same place are their direct descendants. More challenging antigen tests might reveal specific disease antibodies, showing which ills PUM II suffered (such as viral hepatitis); this could open the way for immunity profiles of entire ancient populations. It was also hoped that identifying still other families of proteins would tell much about PUM II's nutrition, diet, and general health, and the presence or absence of certain genetic metabolic defects.

Even the simplest of these tests is full of pitfalls. For instance, bacterial contamination can give false blood-type results. It was possible, by using two different tests, to confirm that PUM II belonged to blood type B. The other results were more ambiguous. Some proteins were found, but they had degenerated too much to be identified. Researchers had to hope that better results might come from better lab techniques or better preserved bodies, such as those frozen in Alaskan ice.

Next came what are called neutron activation tests, to learn the concentrations of various metals in PUM II's body. Again there were technical problems, such as contamination by embalming substances, but clearly PUM II's body contained only one-tenth as much lead as our bodies do today, suggesting a dramatic modern increase in environmental lead. Tests of PUM II's muscle tissue revealed zinc deficiency, which still causes anemia and retarded maturation in many young Egyptian males.

All of these findings appeared gradually; the Cockburns and their colleagues published the first facts in a newsletter they bravely called *Paleopathology Newsletter No. 1*, not seriously expecting that a second issue would appear. But PUM II's autopsy caught the imaginations of the press and of scientists all over the world. Letters came from cultural and physical anthropologists, historians, physicians. In 1974 the PUM team had organized the Paleopathology Association, a group with two hundred members in a dozen nations, and they began publishing the newsletter on a regular quarterly basis. Four years later, there were three hundred members in twenty-two nations — among them myself, already a fascinated follower of their progress. Paleopathology, long little more than an idea, was on the way to becoming an interdisciplinary specialty taught in several dozen universities.

When the Cockburns did another autopsy, in 1974, they were able to enlist more than forty specialists. This mummy's coffin gave his name as Nakht and his occupation as weaver at a temple dedicated to the spirit of the pharaoh Setnakht. Nakht hadn't been chosen at random. His coffin showed that he had been a worker who died in Thebes about 3,200 years ago; rarely can one pinpoint a mummy so precisely in time and place. Furthermore, few mummies of people from Nakht's social class have survived; most couldn't afford expensive funerals, let alone mummification. (Nakht's coffin, which cost about a tenth of a year's wages, may have been a fringe benefit for temple workers.) Also, historians know more about Nakht's era than about most others in ancient Egypt — a time of political uncertainty and spiraling inflation when people such as Nakht probably worked hard, ate none too well, and lived in modest homes of mud brick.

Nakht had been washed and wrapped in linen; the dry climate alone preserved him. In life he had been between five foot six and five foot ten and weighed 100 to 120 pounds. X-rays of his skeleton gave his age at death as between fourteen and eighteen; the younger age is more likely, for teeth and bones probably matured a couple of years later in Nakht's time than today. Harris lines tell of severe, recurring illness or malnutrition during his last two years. Nakht's remains, unlike PUM II's, suggest what his fatal ills were.

Nakht's liver and kidneys contained schistosome eggs; the damage they did showed in cirrhosis of the liver, in the bladder, and in blood (the oldest red blood cells ever found in human remains). In fact, Nakht was a veritable museum of parasitic infections. His intestines contained tapeworm eggs, and his spleen seemed enlarged, perhaps ruptured, raising the possibility of malaria. Nakht was subjected to a battery of blood-typing, antibody, and other lab tests. As in PUM II's case, proteins weren't preserved well enough for many to be identified, but there were some rough results. Nuclear medical tests for hepatitis antigen were negative, but tests of spleen tissue for malaria antigens were tentatively positive.

The autopsies of PUM II and Nakht challenged some assumptions about the past and present. Both Egyptians, from different periods and social classes, were ridden by parasites and marked by childhood ills, their harsh desert environment, and less than ideal nutrition. Their entire society may have been sapped by endemic malaria, schistosomiasis, and intestinal parasites; many who survived early adulthood suffered such degenerative diseases as arteriosclerosis and arthritis, which we have tended to associate not only with middle age but with modern living conditions.

Furthermore, the studies of PUM II and Nakht set new standards and introduced new methods. No longer do paleopathologists rapidly autopsy hundreds or thousands of mummies, looking for gross pathology. Now the lab work can take as long as a decade and involve dozens of specialists all over the world. New techniques keep emerging; Nakht was the first mummy to be studied by computerized tomography, or soft-tissue X-ray scanning. Researchers now preserve sample tissues from a mummy autopsy so that they will be available when better techniques appear.

With new techniques, new kinds of information can be sought. Blood-typing may some day help confirm the family relationships among the royal mummies; such studies have already been done on the body of Tutankhamon. More important, the proportions of blood types in a population over time may tell who they were, how they have changed, and whether they have moved geographically. The skulls and teeth of the Nubians suggested that the present-day population are direct, undiluted descendants of the Nubians who lived under the late Egyptian kings.

Attempts to confirm such information by blood-typing go back to the thirties, but recent techniques make them more reliable. Studies of mummies ranging from five hundred to two thousand years old on the Peruvian coast have shown the same proportions of blood types as the Indians who live there today. Immunological studies of Peruvian mummies also confirmed historical assumptions that in certain areas the native population intermarried (or at least interbred) with Spanish colonists. Research of this kind has helped sort out the complicated shifts of several populations in past centuries in Hungary.

With enough information about large populations over long periods, we may even start to understand how blood types evolved, and why. It was long thought that modern man's ancestors contained only the gene for type O blood, and that the AB groups evolved quite recently. Studies of predynastic Egyptian mummies show that the AB types were already common five thousand years ago. We don't know why different peoples have different proportions of blood types; perhaps the genes responsible for various types help in adapting to certain climates, diets, or disease environments. Understanding the evolution of blood types may bring greater knowledge of antigens and the immune system in general, with implications for such matters as resistance to infectious diseases and cancer.

Research on mummies is already confirming certain views on the nature of cancer in our time. Paleopathologists have hunted for cancer in mummies and ancient bones, but with virtually no success. There are two quite different explanations of its rareness. Some say that cancer has increased in recent times, that in fact it is largely a modern disease. Others have claimed that cancer (or the potential for it) may have been common in past eras, but that the ancient incidence is masked for several reasons: in past millennia, most people didn't live long enough to develop cancer; tumors didn't survive mummification well enough to be detectable; bone cancer usually leaves only a defect indistinguishable from other ills. This is a matter of more than theoretical interest; if cancer is truly more common today than in the past, we will benefit from knowing why.

The problem interested Dr. Michael Zimmerman, a pathologist with a degree in anthropology, who became interested in paleopathology when the Cockburns did, and who often worked with them. Zimmerman studied X-ray surveys of mummies in Egypt and Europe and found no firm diagnoses of cancer. He reviewed autopsy findings and discovered only three microscopic diagnoses of tumors in mummies; one was questionable, and two were benign tumors of the skin. In short, he found not one sure diagnosis of cancer in ancient remains. Like any good biohistorian, he suspended conclusions until he had checked out the potential arguments against his findings.

As a pathologist, Zimmerman routinely performed autopsies on people who had died of a wide variety of diseases. In the course of his work, he took samples of normal and cancerous tissue from every major type of tissue in the body. Then, in an experiment that took many months, he put these tissues through a process that simulated mummification, rehydrated them, and studied them under the microscope. Preservation was a bit better than in real mummies, but the changes were essentially the same. In fact, Zimmerman found that cancerous tissue was actually better preserved than normal tissue. It is not true, then, that mummification masked cancerous cell changes; to the contrary, it enhanced them.

Zimmerman saw holes in several of the arguments that time conceals the existence of cancer in ancient remains. Many people who survived early life in ancient Egypt reached middle or old age; we know that they lived long enough to develop arthritis, arteriosclerosis, and heart attacks, which is the age when cancer starts becoming common. Since surgery and other treatments were not available, a cancer should remain in the mummy of a person who developed it. Finally, although cancer is primarily a disease of later life, leukemia and bone cancer are most common in the first few decades, they haven't been found in the remains of children and adolescents of past eras.

There is also historical evidence. Although Greek physicians described cancer some two thousand years ago, they didn't say it was common, and many kinds of cancer were described for the first time only during the past two centuries. Many of the recently discovered varieties are occupational, caused by exposure to chemicals or irritants. And it was only in the early twentieth century that scientists began to perceive an increase of cancer throughout the world.

Zimmerman's final argument is his own experience. He has carried out autopsies of over a hundred mummies from Egypt, Peru, and Alaska — more, perhaps, than any other person working in paleopathology today. He has discovered not one cancer of the lung, breast, bowel, or any of the other kinds so common today. In our time, about one American in three or four will develop some form of cancer; the disease accounts for 17 percent of all deaths. And it is now believed that as many as three-quarters of all cancers are caused, directly or in part, by tobacco, industrial pollution, radiation, and perhaps by changes in diet, hereditary patterns, and continually evolving viruses. The logical conclusion is that we don't find cancer in ancient bones and mummies because it used to be far rarer, and the recent increase results from modern environmental conditions and life-styles. This conclusion can't be considered ironclad yet, but it is a powerful lead for future research.

To most people, studying mummies still evokes images of gold gravegoods and bizarre ancient customs. That may now be the least important part of studying ancient remains. Paleopathology has gone beyond diagnosing the individual dead, and it will doubtless keep creating new methods and new questions. It can already go beyond the history of human health and disease and begin to reveal the daily lives of vanished people. As the next chapter will show, our lives need not be described in art and writings to leave a record. They are literally inscribed in our bodies and will remain readable millennia later.

5

Dry Bones

THE UNWRITTEN PAST

THE "great man" approach to history, with its dramas of humanity's heroes and monsters, has been falling from fashion for more than a century. The powerful, gifted, and villainous are no less intriguing, but the social and biological sciences have expanded enormously, offering new views of societies and the human species. They make compelling arguments for both continuity and change in human history regardless of the acts of individuals. Besides, there has always been curiosity about how ordinary people lived in the past. This curiosity rises partly from a personal tickle of the imagination: how would I have walked and talked, worked and played, fought and loved, had I lived in Penn's wilderness, the Inca kingdom, or a Neanderthal cave? The farther back one looks in time, the more one must turn to biohistory for answers.

It is relatively easy to learn about daily life in historical periods, chiefly from chronicles and memoirs; searching for Penn's America, the biohistorian uses physical evidence largely to verify and expand on written sources. Looking back to the Egyptians and Incas, he interweaves physical findings with business and government records, temple inscriptions, pictures of religious and legendary figures. The biohistorian's strongest, almost exclusive province has been prehistory, yet only recently could he use physical evidence alone to reveal the ways of people who left little or no record but their bones.

This sort of biohistory offers no narratives like the lives of Napoleon, Poe, or even nameless mummies. Rather, it presents pictures of eras, societies, and our evolving species. To do so, it must plunge into provinces the medical biographer can ignore, coordinating the highly detailed puzzle-solving of specialists who rarely work together. Through a wide array of new ideas and techniques, it has begun to illuminate life in a pre-Columbian kingdom or a long-vanished tribe of nomadic hunters. That it extracts so much knowledge from so little material is one of biohistory's great fascinations.

Unfortunately, the former lack of these concepts and techniques didn't keep people from claiming to reconstruct the past; the results were often a mixture of guesswork and cliché. For instance, illustrations and museum displays routinely show a half-dozen Neanderthalers from ages three to thirty, the women squatting and the men hulking about a fire, all gazing numbly at the middle distance. Films have them grunting, snarling, and constantly trying to brain each other over meat and mates. Actually, it was sheer speculation whether they lived in families or larger groups, how long they lived, how violent and how cooperative they were, which tasks were men's or women's, even whether they sat or squatted. It was assertion, not fact, that they never frolicked with joy, paled in grief, or showed subtler emotions — in short, that they were less expressive than normal baboons.

This lumpish vision of early man was probably inadvertent. Not sure how Neanderthalers felt and acted, art-

ists and anthropologists left a blank where normal life
should be; they may also have presumed a Hobbesian
brutishness in any predecessor of the Victorian upper
classes. Their claylike picture was automatically repeated.
Similar mental habits have shaped conceptions of other
ancient peoples. For instance, we don't know what the
worshippers at Stonehenge looked like, but illustrators
regularly serve up crowds of Celts in animal skins with
ferocious or dreamy expressions, and a white-bearded druid
gazing in wild inspiration at the stars. We don't really
know that a passionate Erse night preceded the Celtic
Twilight, that dolmen builders were never cloddish, druids
never bald, beardless, and serene. Compare pictures of
Amerindians millennia before Columbus, usually shown
tanning skins and weaving baskets with a prosaic air. They
may have had their own passionate myths and magic, and
Celts surely did the same prosaic labors, but few pictures
make you think so.

The biohistorian must reach beyond such inherited visions. Much will always be inference, but now he can verify
more than ever before, by using the tools and interdisciplinary teamwork described in the previous chapter for
studying mummies. He combines the expanding reaches
of anthropology, archaeology, chemistry, clinical medicine, pathology, ethology, sociobiology, and paleobotany.
The work is so new and challenging that no cultural re-
construction has yet used all of these new resources. We
will look at a number of them and suggest how they can
be combined, as they doubtless will be soon.

As in the past, the task will usually start with human
bones; sometimes they are all the biohistorian has to work
with. Unearthing ancient bones strikes most people as a
romantic calling, studying them a dry one. By unfortunate
coincidence, anthropologists and pathologists themselves

distinguish ancient skeletal remains from recent ones by the term "dry bones." But now dry bones can reveal stories imprinted on them millennia ago, allowing us to put one foot in vanished peoples' villages and campsites, and sometimes even to enter their minds.

The simplest messages in bones beyond people's size, physique, and facial contours are their life spans and peaks of mortality (the ages at which deaths are most common). Recent studies refute some old assumptions on even such basic matters. Scientists long assumed that recent pre-technological peoples reflected human life everywhere five thousand and fifty thousand years ago. In most places they saw high infant mortality and short life spans, so they assumed that life throughout prehistory was universally brutish and brief, with many infants born and many dying, and most adults perishing early of violence or disease. Now dry bones show that this assumption reached too far.

Scientist Steven Clarke recently compared the bones of five prehistoric peoples from Nubia, Illinois, and Arizona; in all five, infant mortality was lower than in many poor societies today. The peaks of mortality were at ages two to six and twenty to thirty; life was apparently most threatening after weaning, probably by nutritional stress, and in early adulthood, by hunting, combat, and childbearing. Still, there were individuals who survived both periods of life, and researchers have found a number of skeletons from Saxon England and even the Neanderthal age, some fifty thousand years ago, that reveal life spans of forty or fifty years.

These and other studies over the past two decades have shown that life span and mortality peaks varied widely among ancient societies. For instance, the bones of Indians living in Ohio a thousand years ago reveal both short life spans and low infant mortality; the reason is yet to be learned. Some paleopathologists think the short life and high infant mortality so common in recent nonwestern societies came chiefly from exposure to European diseases and from colonial changes in living conditions. Apparently health and longevity have varied in complex ways because of changes in technology, social organization, the environment, and the microbes that coexist with man.

Bones also reveal the kind and extent of violence in societies, a matter that involves our basic view of human nature. There has been passionate dispute about whether aggression is part of our genetic inheritance or a result of social forces and individual experience. Much of the heat comes from biological determinists, who see people only as expressions of a gene pool, and from social determinists, who speak as if people were astral bodies. The biohistorian, grounded in both social and biological science, must take a middle ground: violence is a universal human potential, cultivated by some societies and minimized by others.

It is now widely accepted that a couple of million years ago, prehuman primates used stones to smash the bones of animals, and perhaps each other, to extract the marrow. Some even claim that tool-using and violence evolved together. Certainly there is massive evidence from ethology (the study of animal behavior) and sociobiology (the study of the genetic roots of behavior) that violence has been part of our evolutionary heritage over millions of years. Confirmation comes from the skeletal record of violence through prehistory. During the first half of this century, a small number of anthropologists and doctors tried to read that record in ancient bone fractures, with varying success. Their successors have refined diagnostic and statistical methods and reached firmer conclusions.

Once it was thought that an animal with a broken bone, unable to hunt or defend itself, would soon die, and that this was true of early man as well. However, researchers have found well-healed fractures in wild gorillas and chimps and in our hominid ancestors. It is no surprise, then, to find them in early humans; in fact, what demands explanation is their very great number. This requires that the biohistorian become a coroner solving very tricky problems of discrimination. A bone may have been broken after death, by humans or earth movements or the pressure of growing tree roots. A crushing skull wound or broken ribs may have resulted from a blow, fall, or rockslide. A missing limb may have been severed in battle, as legal punishment, or even by medical amputation, which the Egyptians used to treat crushing injuries four thousand years ago and perhaps earlier.

Biohistorians have found ingenious ways to choose among such explanations. A fracture marks a bone indelibly, and so does healing. If a break shows no healing, we know it happened no earlier than a week before death. If an arm was severed and the person survived, the collarbone and shoulder blade eventually undergo a characteristic atrophy. The blows of a stone ax, arrow tip, rock from a sling, and metal blade all have specific signatures. Even defense leaves its own signs on the bones. When someone reflexively raises an arm to deflect a blow to the head, the result is a "parry fracture" of the forearm. The great majority of people, being right-handed, wield a weapon with the right arm and defend themselves with the left; therefore the majority of blows land on an opponent's left side and forearm. Doubt may remain about the bones of any individual, but the number, kind, and location of fractures in a population are decisive. If many individuals have fractures of the left forearm and the left side of the skull and body, the society was obviously more combative than accident-prone.

Evidence has accumulated through dozens of studies not only that violence abounded in early societies, but that many people survived it for years and decades. There are many healed fractures caused by rocks or clubs in the skulls of Java man and Peking man, hundreds of thousands of years ago. Puncture wounds, perhaps made by something like a pickax, occur in the skulls of Rhodesian man and other Paleolithic (Old Stone Age) peoples. The very first Neanderthaler ever discovered, in 1856, had what looks like a healed parry fracture. Virtually every complete Neanderthal skeleton, and almost half of Neanderthal skulls, bear marks of injury, many by hafted stone axes.

A painstaking study of Neanderthal skeletons has been made by the same Dr. Michael Zimmerman who contributed to research on Egyptian mummies. He examined the bones of seven Neanderthal adults and two infants, about fifty to sixty thousand years old, that had been found in the 1950s in Shanidar Cave in Iraq. Four of the six relatively complete skeletons bore severe injuries, and two of the men were probably crippled by their wounds. One man reached age thirty-five to fifty, having survived multiple fractures of the skull, legs, hands, and feet, and a crushing fracture over the left eye that deformed his face. The wounds may well have left him partially paralyzed on one side and blind in one eye. Some of the injuries may have resulted from accidents, but hardly all. Whatever their cause, he could have reached middle age only if he received much nursing and help over several periods of his life. Obviously Neanderthalers didn't just cast aside the wounded, disabled, and aging, a fact as important as their pugnacity.

The record of violence and survival continues in Cro-Magnon skulls of the Paleolithic age. Neolithic (New Stone Age) bones of the New and Old Worlds also bear the healed head wounds, parry fractures, and hand fractures of close combat. From the later Neolithic on, violent injuries started increasing in number and severity. Bones from early historic Egypt and Rome show violence and technology growing together; metal weapons made more skull wounds fatal, more body blows crippling. The trend was to continue; a study of skeletons in Greece from 6500 B.C. to modern times reveals fractures in ever-growing numbers. Violence then grew by staggering progressions with the development of explosives, firearms, and nuclear weapons, culminating in this century with the maiming and killing of tens of millions of people in each of several decades.

Prehistory and early history weren't times of universal, unremitting violence. Then, as today, some societies were less combative than others. For instance, there are few smashed skulls, hacked limbs, and parry fractures in Neolithic bones unearthed near Loisy, in France. The same signs of a relatively peaceful life appear in bones from medieval cemeteries in Normandy and York. American anthropologists who recently studied Indians of the Late Woodland period (about A.D. 1000) in Ohio found few combat fractures, and determined that injuries occurred steadily over individuals' lives. This suggests the gradual toll of labor and accidents, not fits of battle.

One traditional view of humanity, bolstered by simplistic Darwinism, paints nature red in tooth and claw, and boasts that civilization tamed the human beast. Rousseauistic, backward-looking utopians have asserted the contrary; they portray early humans as a pastoral crafts colony turned to snarling by private property, plumbing, and the multiplication table. Both views violate the bio-historian's evidence that humans as a species have always been more or less aggressive, but with important variations in how much, to whom, and why.

The old Latin tag says that man is a wolf to man. One can only wish it were true, for deadly infraspecies violence is not wolfish but peculiarly human. As Konrad Lorenz and other ethologists have shown, wolves are highly aggressive, like all territorial, predatory creatures; but like all such creatures, especially those that live in groups, they have developed efficient aggression controls, from ritual-ized combat to a rather stable dominance system. After all, survival means not only hunting but mutual defense, cooperation, mating, and raising the young. Wolves' fights end in surrender, not death, and most aggression is among males, not by males against weaker females and young.

Humans, like wolves, evolved as social, predatory, ter-ritorial creatures. Because of children's uniquely pro-longed helplessness, humans have also had to be especially cooperative and nurturing. Therefore it isn't strange that Neanderthalers fought so much and nursed their wounded so tenaciously, nor that most combat fractures are in adult males. Furthermore, most societies roughly mirror the wolf pack's restraints on aggression. Virtually every peo-ple have customs and laws that discourage and punish unlimited or random mayhem.

Consider, though, the site of a fortified village at Crow Creek, South Dakota, on a bluff over the Missouri River, studied recently by a team of doctors and anthropologists. There, in the fourteenth century, some five hundred men, women, and children were buried together. Unhealed fractures were rife, the heads, hands, and feet had been severed from many bodies, and the majority of skulls bear the scratches typical of scalping. Very few of the fractures were defensive. It seems that a whole village of poeple were sneaked up on, captured, massacred, mutilated, and dumped in the moat that had failed to protect them.

Such behavior shows a terrible gulf between humans and any comparable species. If people were truly as wolves to each other, they would kill only to eat and rarely harm each other beyond occasional bullying and beating. Humans are the only higher social species that kill their own in great numbers, including females and the young. Now biohistorians' research shows that this lethal infraspecies aggression has increased over time. The explanation, I suggest, lies in the same source as the growth of civilization itself — the expansion of technology and the varieties of cultures.

Homicide wasn't easy for the earliest men; the decisive leap in aggression may have occurred not with hand-held weapons or firearms but with the first long-distance weapons. It is difficult to kill a person with one's bare hands, easier with a club, still easier with a pike or sword. But human life must have changed irrevocably when the bow and slingshot first allowed killing from a distance.* Firearms made killing still easier and less personal. In our century, dropping bombs and firing missiles merely extended a trend that began tens of thousands of years ago. Like the five-part fugue, molecular chemistry, and the practice of biohistory, violence expanded with the use of

---

*Today the slingshot is a toy, but a trained slinger is lethal from afar. The Romans and other ancient peoples had legions of them, and their ammunition left unmistakable marks on enemies' skulls. The effects of javelins and bows and arrows are less conclusive because these, unlike slingshot projectiles, are often deadly without damaging bones.

the cerebral cortex. The cortex performs problem-solving and leaps of invention, but it does not direct the controls on violence; these reside in the more primitive midbrain.

Technology alone doesn't explain the growth of violence. There is sometimes aggression within families and communities, but it is in fights between societies that limits on violence most dramatically fail. We have become what ethologist Desmond Morris calls a species of tribes and super-tribes, in-groups and out-groups. People who share a territory, language, customs, and beliefs become what I would call a social species, viewing different peoples as different kinds of creatures. Like wolves that protect their own young but slaughter infant deer, humans who cherish their kin and neighbors may butcher foreign men, women, and children.

Social species probably began to multiply and grow in complexity ten thousand years ago, with the shift to agriculture. Through most of their history, humans had probably lived in groups of a few dozen to a few hundred mobile hunter-gatherers. With the emergence of agriculture, cities, and nations, they began to perceive their social species as comprising not just a small band but simultaneously a region, nation, religion, class, caste, race, political faction. Now the main thrust of human evolution was not physical but cultural. This profusion of tribes, subtribes, and supertribes created more and more situations in which people violently excluded each other from nature's usual rules of infraspecies coexistence.

Paradoxically, the very technology that spawned so much depersonalized violence also preserved and enhanced life. Professor Ralph Solecki of Columbia University, who unearthed the Shanidar skeletons, found with them the pollen of clusters of medicinal herbs, which apparently were known and gathered by Neanderthalers. As the ways of smashing bones improved, so did ways of mending them. One can't always be sure whether a prehistoric fracture was treated, but many apparently were. The bonesetter's art is old, in some societies distinct from that of other healers; it is practiced quite well by many pretechnological peoples today, by setting, immobilization, traction, and massage. More dramatic still are the many ancient skulls that show successful trepanation, the removal of a piece of skull to expose the brain. This operation was common in Europe ten thousand years ago and continued into the Middle Ages; it was quite widely done in Peru a couple of thousand years ago. Trepanation was probably first performed to relieve pressure on the brain by blood and bone after crushing skull wounds; some societies have also used it to treat headaches, epilepsy, and mental illness.

Such surgery was done in the past as it is today in Bolivia and Kenya, drilling or scraping the skull with flint tools until a piece can be removed. Alcohol or coca may be used as anesthetic, and the task efficiently performed within hours. In some societies, the recovery rate has been well over 50 percent. There are Neolithic skulls showing several trepanations, even a half dozen, all of which healed without infection.

We have now found several points on which the usual picture of prehistoric people should be revised. Some of them should be forty or fifty, and one of the men scarred, even crippled, by accidents and battle wounds. He could be lying with a nasty wound on the left side of his head and a broken left forearm, carefully nursed by a relative or friend. Perhaps the broken bone is even being set. If one of the men is to be shown fighting, which isn't a bad idea, it should probably be with someone from a neighboring band, not from his own group. Individuals shouldn't be expressionless or standing without relation to each other;

their expressions and gestures should suggest a close-knit, cooperative group. Should they be sitting, kneeling, squatting, standing, or sprawled on the ground? Sometimes we can answer this apparently minor point, which opens the door to very important ones.

In people who habitually squat on their heels, the facets of certain foot bones flatten; kneeling causes similar but distinguishable changes. "Squatting facets" have been found in Copper Age skeletons in France, so one should portray those people squatting at work or rest. Like most skeletal evidence, squatting facets require a careful search for alternative explanations. What look like squatting facets may result from a lifetime of walking on rough, mountainous terrain; the giveaway is severe wear and tear of the heels and knees. Such a combination of changes appears in the bones of the ancient Palomans of Peru, some six thousand years ago. We cannot be sure whether they squatted or only had what resembled squatting facets because they spent their lives climbing Andean slopes. In ancient skeletons from Equador, kneeling facets are more marked in women than men; probably both sexes knelt at rest, and women knelt at their daily tasks as well. Their bones hint at not only habitual postures but one of the most important features of any society, its daily work and the sexual division of labor. The study of fractures, arthritis, and other bone changes tell more.

The heavy use of any joint can eventually cause not only fractures but a variety of degenerative changes laymen lump together under the term arthritis. Arthritis appears most in the spine and limbs, which take the strain of weight-bearing and heavy or repetitive labor, and it varies by age, sex, genetic susceptibility, and work patterns. Furthermore, bones accommodate to the overdevelopment of muscles attached to them, producing subtle signs of sustained, specialized work. Today there are predictable bone changes in the hands of crop pickers, the backs of lumberjacks, and the knees of miners. Similar changes testify to ancient peoples' labors. A man buried by the eruption of Vesuvius nineteen hundred years ago, a sword by his side, had arm bones enlarged by years of carrying a shield in one hand and throwing a javelin with the other, and knees adapted to a horseman's muscles. If we hadn't already known that the Romans had a professional military, including cavalry, we would have learned it from his bones.

Bones now give an especially interesting picture of labor and life-styles before, during, and after the transition from hunting and gathering to agriculture — the "agricultural revolution" from which modern society and technology arose. The anthropological truism is that men hunt and women gather, and so it doubtless was for hundreds of thousands of years. Recent research makes this more than speculation. For instance, in the bones of pre-Columbian Indians on the California coast, men's most common bone traumas were parry fractures. Most common in women were Colles' fractures, breaks in the ankle that come from slipping on rough terrain. Clearly the men hunted and fought, and the women gathered shellfish on the slippery rocks by the sea.

Arthritic changes also speak clearly about the shift in labor that came with changes in subsistence. Hunter-warriors suffer combat wounds, accidents, and, since men everywhere do the tasks demanding peak strength, traumas such as "fatigue fractures" of the lower vertebrae, the cracking of bone under stress. One would also expect the use of spears, bows, and other weapons to strain the wrist and shoulder and cause injuries similar to tennis elbow and pitcher's arm. There are indeed marks of com-

bat, weapon use, and peak effort on prehistoric male skeletons all over the world, from Greece to Brazil. Women
did the less intense but more sustained labor of digging,
carrying, and preparing food and hides, tasks that put
chronic wear on the fingers and elbows.

When anthropologist Robert Pickering studied the bones
of ancient hunter-gatherers in Illinois, he found arthritic
changes reflecting just such work patterns in men and
women, and an interesting age difference as well. Arthritis
was worst at women's elbows and thumbs, and it appeared
in the mid-twenties. Men eventually suffered more arthritis, especially at the wrists and elbows, but it began a
few years later. The age difference makes sense if one
recalls that labor-related arthritis may take a decade to
develop, and that boys and girls reach social maturity at
different ages. The people Pickering studied probably lived
like such modern hunter-gatherers as the !Kung of Africa:
the girls start to gather and perform other female chores
at fourteen, but boys don't become hunters till sixteen or
older. This fits biological expectations; in humans, as in
many higher species, females reach physical and social
maturity before males.

Hunter-gatherers of both sexes suffered many fractures
and arthritic changes compared to modern city dwellers.
Those in the harshest environments, such as Eskimos, had
very high rates of degenerative joint disease and fatigue
fractures at early ages. The skeletal record shows that the
transition to agriculture first made life dramatically easier
and healthier in many parts of the world. For instance,
the pathology of bones from Neolithic France differs little
from that of modern Americans. But eventually agriculture brought complex changes in labor, life-style, and health,
and not all were for the better.

One obvious change was the shift to intensive farm labor

itself. In some places, where villages grew into cities, there was a specialization of labor among farmers, soldiers, and such sedentary classes as craftsmen, tradesmen, clergy, and even idle rich. But for the great majority of people, the agricultural revolution meant full-time farming, which is correctly called backbreaking work even today. Both sexes became chained to hard, sustained, repetitive labor. To grasp what it was like, a modern city dweller should spend a numbing day with a hoe or scythe and imagine doing it with a wooden plow or a sickle with a blade of flint chips. Many European bones from the late Neolithic until recent times show severe work damage to the lower back and limbs, almost enough to have made farmers nostalgic for mammoth hunting and roving territorial skirmishes.

It is still possible for a world traveler to see firsthand the myriad, profound differences between a nomadic band, a small farm village, and a city. The agricultural revolution and urban growth must have touched every daily detail of social, economic, and political life. Larger, settled populations offered wider choices of mates and underwent genetic changes. Shifts in the division of labor may have affected property and inheritance laws, sex roles, family life, child rearing. Research and debate continue about these matters as we observe them in this century; we can only guess about the past. But ingenious collaborative studies keep adding to our knowledge. Now this can be done when people didn't even leave their bones to posterity; we can know them through their debris.

A good example is a study by a score of specialists in a cave near the coast of northern Spain, where huntergatherers camped for twelve thousand years, starting twentyone thousand years ago. No human bones remained, but scientists went through layers of debris, identifying thousands of fragments of animal bones, mollusc shells, and tools. First, paleontologists determined the kinds and proportions of animals, fish, and shellfish as they changed along with the local vegetation and climate. Then the research turned to paleobotany, the study of ancient plants and pollens, which has become a well-developed specialty over the past sixty years. Pollen, unlike plants, is preserved rather easily, and that of each species is distinctive. At the Spanish cave, paleobotanists gathered pollen from the floor layer by layer, classified, counted, and thus reconstructed the region's flora over twelve thousand years. Changes in the flora allowed them to deduce changes in the total environment, from weather to the food chain.

It became clear that changing technology had helped hunter-gatherers to broaden their diets. The appearance of bones from saltwater fish told when they began using fish traps or nets. Bits of bone harpoons showed when they started hunting large sea creatures. We have yet to learn whether subsistence technology developed with a momentum of its own, because old food sources dwindled or changed, because of population pressures, or because a kinder climate offered new opportunities. We do know from such research that the agricultural revolution was not an unprecedented stroke of invention; for millennia many hunter-gatherers had used better tools to broaden their diets. Whatever the reason, people in many parts of the world began herding wild animals and eventually bred these into new domesticated species, and they started planting grains instead of gathering them from the wild.

There were obvious advantages in turning to agriculture. Hunter-gatherers' bones show that sometimes they had good and varied diets, but sometimes fell prey to the changing bounty of the seasons and the environment. In temperate climates, they often suffered from winter bouts of protein deficiency, scurvy, and famine. We noted in the previous chapter that so-called Harris lines appear in a young person's bones when growth resumes after a period of illness or malnutrition; a Harris line's distance from the end of the bone tells when it was laid down. Both well-nourished and chronically malnourished people show few Harris lines; the former have little to recover from, the latter rarely recover fully. But people who experience periodic ills or deprivations show many Harris lines, and that is what one finds in many hunter-gatherers. Such lines were once numerous, for instance, in the bones of Indians in California; they decreased when the people learned to store acorns, providing themselves with important vitamins and minerals during the winters.

There is confirmation of this in the so-called Wilson's bands in tooth enamel. Like Harris lines, they reflect illness or stress in the growing years, but they result from the insult to the body, not from renewed growth afterward. Wilson's bands don't always correspond precisely with Harris lines, but they are a good rough guide to health and nutrition. They are especially good indicators of weanling disease, the often fatal diarrhea and vulnerability to infection that strike children who stop nursing and try to adapt to an inadequate diet.

Early farmers may have imagined a future of unending and universal plenty. Ancient bones and teeth show that agriculture's changes weren't all for the better; in fact, the effects on nutrition were sometimes devastating. This was primarily because of overdependence on cereals that are high in carbohydrates and calories but low in protein. One of the most striking changes in ancient skeletons is a decrease in many peoples' height after the advent of agriculture. For instance, skeletons from ancient Greece show a decrease in size seven thousand years ago, when the

Paleolithic diet of meat and plants gave way to a diet high in cultivated cereal; height improved with the return to a more varied diet five thousand years later. Carbohydrates also took a high toll in tooth decay and root abscesses. Caries increased greatly in Peru four thousand years ago, with a shift from fishing to farming; the absence of caries in Equador at the same time is enough to make biohistorians infer that agriculture still wasn't intensive there.

Harris lines, Wilson's bands, and caries all increased dramatically in Amerindians who depended heavily on maize. This has become indisputable only over the past decade, and it has helped to clarify a half-century of disputes about one of history's longstanding puzzles, the fall of the Maya empire. Back in 1930, the eminent Harvard anthropologist Earnest Hooton published a study of Maya remains at Chichén Itzá, in Yucatan. There he had found skeletons dating from about A.D. 900–1200, the time of the empire's rapid decline. In two-thirds of the children between six and twelve, Hooton had found pitting of the orbital bones and a spongy change in the cranium called osteoporosis (or, more recently, porotic hyperostosis). Hooton went on to compare the Maya skulls with those of modern children suffering a genetic anemia called thalassemia. He saw a similarity and guessed in 1940 that "osteoporosis caused the downfall of Maya civilization."

This joined a long list of alleged causes for the Maya decline — revolution, invasion, malaria, soil exhaustion, crop failures, a population outgrowing its food supply. There was no decisive proof for or against any of these until paleopathologists' studies began to multiply a few decades later. Only in recent years do they allow a firm answer to Hooton's guess.

First, several possibilities can be eliminated, including Hooton's. Pitted orbits and hyperostosis do occur in the

Old World because of malaria and genetic anemias such as sickle-cell disease and thalassemia. However, thalassemia is usually fatal in early childhood, and the sickle-cell trait and malaria probably reached the New World for the first time with African slaves, centuries after the Mayan downfall. Therefore none of these ills can explain the pathology of Maya skulls, let alone the fall of the empire.

Physicians, anthropologists, and historians are now rather certain, as Hooton could not be, that the commonest cause of pitted orbits and hyperostosis is iron-deficiency anemia. The ultimate reason may be too little iron in the diet, inability to absorb it in the intestine, loss of iron in blood and sweat, or anything that interferes with iron metabolism and hemoglobin formation. Even in purely dietary cases, iron deficiency alone isn't usually the answer; poor nutrition is rarely that selective. People who lack iron may also lack the vitamin C the body needs to absorb and use iron or the protein required for hemoglobin synthesis. Anemia and its effects on the bones often accompany rickets, scurvy, and other signs of poor general nutrition.

Pitting of the orbits, now thought to be a precursor of hyperostosis of the skull vault, has been found in malnourished children throughout history. It struck almost all the Jewish children who hid and starved in caves two thousand years ago during the Roman sieges of the war of Bar Kochba. It was common in ancient Nubia, where the soil is very poor in iron. It is widespread today near the equator, where heavy sweating causes high iron loss, and parasitic infections such as hookworm and tapeworm produce chronic intestinal bleeding. In some places, it appears with weanling diarrhea; the mother's milk is low in iron, and the switch to a diet still poorer in iron makes anemia acute.

In Mexico and Guatemala today there are Indians of unmixed Maya descent, and studies of their health and customs show that they are subject to virtually every kind of iron deficiency. The soil is poor in iron, and so is mothers' milk. Weanling diarrhea is rife, as it was in the past; Spanish colonists recorded that the Maya weaned their children at three or four, and ancient Maya teeth show heavy Wilson's bands at that age. Intestinal parasites take a dreadful toll in illness and death, especially among children. People sweat heavily in the hot, damp climate. Perhaps worst of all, the modern Mayas' diet is very like their ancestors'.

Modern and ancient Maya alike depended heavily on the maize and beans they grew; both are low in proteins, high in carbohydrates. There is almost no vitamin C in the Maya diet, and they cook their food for a long time in water, destroying most of the folic acid and vitamin B_{12} needed for developing red blood cells. Corn contains iron, but it also contains phytic acid, which inhibits iron absorption in the intestine. Now research suggests that the traditional grinding of corn with stones also has the ultimate effect of chemically inhibiting iron absorption.

Scientists have now studied thousands of historic and prehistoric Indian skulls from all over the New World; hyperostosis caused by anemia is clearly higher where people became dependent on maize. Severe anemia struck the Maya, and their environment and customs added to the problem. This was not an affliction that hit them suddenly; Maya body size had decreased a thousand years before the empire disintegrated. Perhaps invasion or social and political upheavals did reduce their great alliance of city-states to scattered, impoverished villages, but the people had long been stunted and weakened by a shift to a drastically unbalanced agricultural diet.

Research on the Maya is only one example of how new information about ancient peoples is coming over the horizon with advancing knowledge and technology in chemistry and physiology. Since the sixties, biohistorians have been measuring with increasing accuracy skeletal trace elements, those minerals that occur in the bones in minute amounts. The results help reveal ancient diet and subsistence patterns, because certain elements are more plentiful in some foods than in others. Such research demands sophisticated laboratory analysis, and interpretation remains difficult. Some minerals don't accumulate in the bones; others can be absorbed after death from the soil; minerals interact in the body in ways not fully understood. Still, some very educated guesses have become possible through recent research.

It seems that when people change from a varied plant diet to heavy dependence on cereals, their bones show an increase in copper and a decrease in zinc. Cadmium is plentiful in molluscs and crustaceans from the sea, but in few other foods, and the bones absorb it. Such knowledge is being put to use in a team study of the ancient Palomans, who adapted from hunting and gathering to agriculture on the Peruvian coast five to seven thousand years ago. The trace elements in their bones suggest a gradual change to cereal and a continued dependence on shellfish. Some Paloman natural mummies survive, and studies are being made of trace elements in their hair; as in the study of Napoleon's alleged poisoning, hairs are cut into many sections to discover the metal's intake over time — in this case, to see if there were seasonal variations. The metal strontium appears in different amounts in Paloman men and women, as it does in meats and plants, suggesting differences in their diets. Further knowledge will come from new techniques for analyzing traces of blood on im-

plements six thousand years or more old and identifying
the animals from which they came. This sort of research
may eventually show dietary and other differences within
societies over time and among sexes, age groups, and
social classes. Recent research on prehistoric Indians in
Tennessee has revealed greater height and trace-element
signs of better nutrition in skeletons found in higher-status
burial sites.

Other discoveries are rising from new scientific instruments. Dr. Alan Walker of Johns Hopkins University has
found that the scanning electron microscope reveals typical patterns of wear on ancient teeth caused by eating
grasses, leaves, fruit, and other kinds of food. (It may also
add to evidence that protohumans used chipping and cutting tools more than two million years ago.) Researchers
at the University of Massachusetts have taken advantage
of the fact that the antibiotic tetracycline is absorbed by
bone and, under certain conditions, shows as yellow flu-
orescence under ultraviolet light. They have discovered
tetracycline in the bones of Sudanese Nubians from almost
two thousand years ago. Tetracycline, like penicillin, is
produced naturally by a microbe that flourishes in damp
cereal; these streptomyces are the commonest bacteria in
Nubian soil. Apparently the Nubians stored grain, providing an ideal environment for streptomyces, and accidentally ate enough natural tetracycline to have received
a therapeutic effect.

Genetics and clinical medicine may eventually allow
inferences about ancient peoples' social structures and
marriage customs. This is possible because of greater understanding of the genetic susceptibility underlying a high
incidence of cleft palate, spina bifida (a severe congenital
defect of the spine), and some two dozen other skeletal
defects and disorders. A very high incidence of spina bifida

has been found in the bones of the vanished Modoc Indians of the American Northwest and in an isolatd prehistoric people in Morocco. Other congenital bone malformations were common in Neolithic France. It is now safe to assume that these findings reflect a rather high degree of inbreeding, the marriage of genetically related people over an extended period.

Sometimes there are more subtle skeletal signs of inbreeding. The Merovingians of southern Germany, around A.D. 500–725, suffered many disorders of the hips, knees, and elbows. Today such problems usually result from violence and heavy labor, and are more common in men than in women. Among the Merovingians, they were common in both sexes; this hints at a genetic susceptibility in the entire population, which suggests inbreeding.

Such evidence raises matters as basic to humanity as violence, labor, subsistence, and kinship. Every society has rules of exogamy, promoting marriage outside one's own social group (defined variously as one's family, village, tribe, clan, caste, or social class). Exogamy reduces inbreeding's risk of harmful genetic traits and acts as a sort of social cross-fertilization. In the ancient Moroccans and Merovingians, did inbreeding result from physical isolation? Isolation through conflicts with neighboring peoples? Harmful social customs? It remains for anthropologists and paleopathologists to collaborate in answering such questions and re-create ancient patterns of family structure, other social structures, and marriage customs. They will probably start most easily by studying genetic defects in early historical peoples, of whose customs there are written records, or people such as the Maya, of whom we have physical and written records from ancient to modern times, and extrapolating backward.

There is still another new source of knowledge about

ancient peoples who did not even leave their bones — the
study of coprolites, or fossilized dung. These survive abun-
dantly in old cesspits in northwestern Europe and in arid
regions such as the American West and Southwest. This
subject, which sometimes needs all the help it can get, is
freshened by the names of some of the places where coprolites are found, such as Dirty Shame Rockshelter in
Oregon, Danger Cave in Utah, and Devil's Lair in western
Australia. Such sites have yielded coprolites of horses and
mammoths from fifty thousand years ago and humans from
thirty thousand years ago.

The first important studies of coprolites were made in
the early 1940s by a researcher named A. Szidat, who
found eggs of the helminth parasite in feces in the guts
of bog mummies in East Prussia. Other researchers followed his lead and created the new specialty or paleoparasitology. They have examined feces in ancient salt
mines in the Austrian Alps and learned that workers
there two thousand years ago were so heavily infected
by intestinal parasites that they must have often been
doubled over in pain. Others have found pinworm and
tapeworm in human coprolites ten thousand years old in
Danger Cave.

Around 1970, researchers became interested in studying
coprolites for plant fibers, undigested seeds, and fragments of bone and shell, which reveal diet and subsistence
patterns. They have done so with success, helping paleobotanists, paleopathologists, and archaeologists recreate
ancient peoples' diets and environments. In coprolites from
Peru dating back almost four thousand years, they have
now found spores of fungi that attacked the local maize
and cotton crops. Using such tools as the scanning electron
microscope, mass spectrometry, and gas chromatography,
they may soon help trace the evolution not only of hu-

manity and its parasites but of humans' crops and crop diseases.

We have not mentioned the best-known sort of evidence from ancient remains, the context in which archaeologists find them. That has been the subject of a number of popular books; many people have already read about how the condition, position, and surroundings of Danish bog mummies show that some were judicially executed, and others were human sacrifices. Fewer, perhaps, are aware of research like that done among the Bonje of northern Ghana. In traditional Bonje society, women were buried facing west, so that the setting sun would warn them it was time to prepare the evening meal; men were buried facing east, so the rising sun would tell them to leave for the fields. With the Bonje's conversion to Islam, both sexes were buried facing east, according to the custom of the new faith. It may be possible to further trace and date the spread of Islam by studying changes in burial practices.

Soon, perhaps, we will take for granted the blending of such traditional archaeological and anthropological studies with the newer methods of biohistory. For instance, this was done in studying the natural mummy of an Inca boy, eight or nine years old at death, discovered in the high Andes of Chile. His clothes showed his high social status and that he was from northern Chile or southern Bolivia, well over a thousand miles away. Paleopathologists found no sign of illness or violence in his body, not one Harris line in his bones. However, there is a vomit stain on his tunic and a very peaceful expression on his face. He must have been one of the children selected at each summer solstice to be sacrificed all over the Inca empire. Inca chronicles say they were drugged with beer and buried alive after being sent on long treks to the places of sacrifice.

Today the radical expansion of traditional history and archaeology is moving faster than it can be widely applied. The number of people using the new biohistory is still small; the work is time-consuming, funds often limited. Still, a few ambitious attempts are in progress to join paleopathology, paleobotany, paleoparasitology, trace-metal studies, and many other specialties in studying ancient remains from Peru and Brazil. The work will take many years to complete, but it may help set new standards in understanding health, diet, labor, and life-style, each distinguished by age, sex, and perhaps other factors.

There is also a wealth of knowledge to be gained from serology, immunology, and other medical studies of ancient populations. These will be especially helpful in learning about human disease, which has evolved along with every other aspect of life. As roving hunters became villagers and then city dwellers, there was probably an increase in infectious diseases, and a shift in mortality peaks. Tuberculosis and many other diseases were probably first acquired from the animals man domesticated, and flourished in the denser populations of growing settlements. Today new drugs, world travel, and the evolution of the microbes that depend on humans to stay alive continue to undergo accelerating changes. It will take a separate chapter to consider which species is more endangered, man or a number of his microscopic fellow travelers on earth.

6

Biocataclysm

PARTNERS IN ILLNESS

$\mathcal{W}$ E deceive ourselves about the nature of illness, for it seems an interruption. Pain and debility overwhelm us; work, play, even normal rest, all cease. We hang at risk, toys of the unforeseen and uncontrollable. In epidemic form, disease interrupts society the same way; at its worst, it is a biological cataclysm rending the social fabric of a town, a continent, sometimes the entire world. A century of research has brought so much cure and control of infection that many people have never shuddered before such biocataclysm. But we are not immune to disease as grand disaster. The threats of old plagues still prowl the world, and new ones are always in the making. Whether the ill is bubonic plague or AIDS, whether the cause seems to be a virus or divine vengeance, people feel the same helplessness, the same disruption and loss.

This is a narrow view of disease, and it sheds little light on nature or on history. Disease is not really an interruption, and only rarely is our relationship with it just intermittent warfare. We and our parasites are constantly readapting to each other in an effort to survive. Although an epidemic is sometimes the result of a biological accident, it is more often an argument in the course of an indissoluble marriage. This becomes clear when one pauses to take the germ's view of illness. To fully understand disease, one must go even further, seeing it as one thread in an ecological network that may include dozens of species, a changing physical environment, and human culture. Then disease truly becomes a meaningful piece of history. Until recently, that was a view most historians deliberately avoided.

Medical historians used to concentrate on listing, dating, and trying to identify ancient plagues; other historians gave only scant, grudging notice to even this rudimentary biohistory. Great plagues have been recorded for at least four thousand years, starting with the ancient Egyptians, Hebrews, Babylonians, and Chinese. For instance, the book of Exodus says that around 1500 B.C., the Egyptians suffered, as Moses had warned, a plague causing "sores that break into pustules on man and beast." Samuel I tells that a few centuries later, the Philistines were struck by a ghastly pestilence after having seized the Hebrews' holy ark; it left them when they returned the ark, spread to the Israelites, and killed more than fifty thousand of them. Biblical scholars have long cited these epidemics and guessed that they were smallpox or any of a dozen other infections, perhaps even diseases no longer known today. Their tentative dates and diagnoses leave no one with a better sense of history.

Even some ancient chroniclers, however, hinted at the vast social and historical implications of disease. In 431 B.C., when Athens reached its highest cultural and political vigor, it entered the long war against Sparta and its Peloponnesian allies. In 430, besieged Athens was struck by a lethal illness that may have traveled there by ship from Egypt. It never harmed the Peloponnesians, but among

Athenians became pandemic — an epidemic that returned in waves. The epidemic seemed to subside but struck again on the ships Pericles sent against the enemy; it may have killed Pericles himself. Finally it left dead as many as a quarter to half of Athens' citizens and soldiers.

Thucydides, who suffered and survived the pestilence, left a detailed description, yet today it can't be named with certainty. It may have been the European debut of typhoid, smallpox, anthrax, or scarlet fever; the symptoms don't quite match any illness known now, but a disease causes different symptoms in a virgin population than in one with some exposure and immune defenses. Another clue that the disease was new to its victims was the high mortality rate. Thucydides said that corpses lay heaped in streets and temples; dogs, birds, and carrion eaters perished with the people; the dying staggered through the streets, seeking water to ease their unquenchable thirst and burning skins. Paupers inherited fortunes from the rich and tried to squander everything at once, "since money and life alike seemed equally ephemeral." People turned to license, lawlessness, even murder, for no one expected to live to reach trial, and "everyone felt that already a far heavier sentence had been passed on him."

This cruel pandemic left Athens crippled and demoralized, rent the city's social and political fabric, and destroyed its sea power. Athens finally fell after twenty-seven years of war, its full grandeur gone forever, changing the course of history in the Mediterranean. Thucydides hinted that the plague was partly to blame. Yet when modern writers try to explain Athens' fall, too few credit the hammer blow of disease as fully as Thucydides, who witnessed the devastation.

In this century, some scholars began giving a few diseases their full places in history. Typhus was among the first, because of its key role in four centuries of European warfare. It killed many of its victims and many of the body lice that transmitted it, which suggests that it was new to both species. Typhus was probably an ancient disease of rats and mice or of their fleas. For reasons we do not know, the typhus germs — rickettsiae, small bacteria with certain viruslike properties — made the adaptive leap of trying to live with humans and their lice.

Typhus was first recognized in Europe in 1490, when it broke out among the soldiers of Ferdinand and Isabella of Spain; the soldiers may have brought it to Europe from Cyprus. In 1526 it so savaged French troops attacking Naples that the army had to give up its siege. Two decades later, Girolamo Fracastoro, the greatest epidemiologist of his time, gave typhus its first, classic description. For several centuries more it scourged armies, slums, and jails, flourishing wherever there were dirt, overcrowding, poverty, and famine.

We said in the first chapter that Napoleon's Grand Army was shattered in Russia in 1812, after almost two decades of stunning successes. Of three hundred thousand men in the main force entering Russia, only ninety thousand reached Moscow, and the chief reason was typhus. Marshal Ney wrote to his wife, "General Famine and General Winter, rather than Russian bullets, have conquered the Grand Army." Biohistorian Frederick Cartwright added that famine, dirt, rain, and lice made the army a staggering victim of General Typhus as well.

Discovering the rickettsiae and their transmission by lice made it possible to combat typhus with soap and insecticides; eventually vaccines and antibiotics offered prevention and cure. Probably only soap and delousing allowed huge armies to wage years of trench warfare through World War I. Even so, the disease killed some two to three million soldiers and spread through Serbia to Russia, where in 1918–1922 it struck twenty to thirty million people, of whom one-tenth died. In 1919 Lenin, confronting civil and foreign wars, famine, and pestilence, declared, "Either socialism will defeat the louse or the louse will defeat socialism." His timing was lucky. It was in the twenties that typhus ceased to be a global threat.

Bacteriologist Hans Zinsser's *Rats, Lice and History* appeared in 1935 and became one of the decade's most popular books. One chapter of this history of typhus was headed, "On the Influence of Epidemic Disease on Political and Military History, and on the Relative Unimportance of Generals." Despite those words, Zinsser still basically treated disease like a big, ugly stone sporadically dropped into the stream of human events. That view remains common. For instance, high-school students know of the great Irish potato famine and its immediate consequences; fewer people know that similar conditions existed in Belgium, Germany, and other parts of Europe during the 1840s; fewer still know of the millions of deaths from typhus that broke out among the malnourished poor, and the role typhus thus played in the Irish and German mass migrations of that era, with effects on the history of the United States, Australia, and other nations.

The first disease to receive its full historical due was the black death, the catastrophic medieval outbreak of the plague — also called bubonic plague, though that is only one form of the disease. The plague's first known devastation of Europe had occurred in 542–548. The Roman empire had split in two; the western part, with its capital in Rome, had fallen, perhaps partly because of epidemics of malaria and other infectious ills. The eastern empire, with its capital in Constantinople, suffered the first brunt of the plague. The disease had left its origins in northeastern India or central Africa, spread to Egypt, and then, perhaps carried by ship rats, it struck the capital of the eastern emperor, Justinian.

The chronicler Procopius left the earliest description of Justinian's plague, as it is still called; it caused swellings, or bubos, in infected lymph glands in the groin, armpits, and neck. It was so devastating, Procopius said, that "the whole human race came near to being annihilated." It must have seemed that way, for in four months it killed two hundred thousand people in Constantinople alone. The disease then scythed through Europe, destroying towns and kingdoms that had been rising from the rubble of the Roman empire. Finally it raged all the way from Ireland and Denmark to Arabia, and perhaps beyond. It did not subside but turned into a pandemic, recurring in cycles of ten to twenty-four years for two centuries.

Modern historians have described some of the ruinous results. In the Near East, North Africa, and Europe, vast die-offs brought civil and agricultural decay; armies trembled and governments fell; Justinian's empire dissolved, to be succeeded by the Byzantine, with its Greek language and culture. The devastation caused the Mediterranean, which had already suffered other pandemics (perhaps virulent measles and smallpox), to lag northern Europe in population and cultural growth for centuries. The Muslim world was also ravaged by the plague; some historians think Islam marched so quickly through so many lands because the plague had preceded it so savagely.

After the plague of Justinian, Europe remained free of serious pandemics for almost a thousand years; the plague become a mention in distant chronicles. Then it hit again in 1347, as part of a worldwide pandemic. It had probably arisen the year before in the Crimea and begun its spread to Scandinavia, Russia, India, China, and Africa. When

Italian traders returned to Genoa from the Middle East, infected rats came on their ships, and the rats' fleas passed the plague to humans. Soon the plague changed from the bubonic to the even more lethal pneumonic form, infecting the lungs and passing directly from person to person by coughing and sneezing.

Only a few days after the plague arrived in Genoa, it began to fly across Italy and the rest of Europe. Petrarch said future generations would not believe such horrors had really happened. Terror of the plague made parents abandon dying children. People facing death indulged in extortion, rape, murder. Boccaccio told of empty houses, abandoned towns, fields and streets littered with corpses, the stink of rotting bodies, a solitude that seemed to dominate the world. Entire ship crews died, and vessels manned only by corpses drifted about the Mediterranean and North Seas.

The black death, as this second plague pandemic was called, may have been the worst cataclysm in humanity's history. It killed well over twenty million people in Europe, a quarter to a third of the continent's population. Tens of thousands of villages were utterly wiped out; many cities lost one-third to two-thirds of their people. The plague killed about a third of Egypt's population and scourged the Middle East, India, and China. Like Justinian's plague, it became a prolonged pandemic; outbursts continued in Europe for three centuries. Its last major appearance in England was the Great Plague of 1665, so brilliantly described in Defoe's *Journal of the Plague Year*. France underwent its last awful epidemic in 1720.

Another surge of the plague occurred in 1896–1904; it killed more than a million people in India, struck Hong Kong and South Africa, and in 1900 touched California. A severe outbreak of the pneumonic form occurred in

Manchuria in 1910–1911. Today antibiotics can combat
the infection; the rats and fleas that carry it can be killed.
Still, the disease has not vanished. It reappeared in Viet-
nam during the war of the 1960s, and in the summer of
1983, dozens of cases appeared in the American Southwest.

The plague has killed more people than any war or
natural disaster, yet for centuries few historians seemed
to appreciate that it changed history accordingly. One
important reason is that disease insults not only individuals
and societies, but historians in particular. It ignores their
theories that great men, masses, or classes shape our destiny. Historians have stood helpless before disease and
seen it as nature's tantrum against humanity, a wrench
thrown into the wheel of "real" history. Lenin acknowl-
edged the power of the louse over the dialectic of class
struggle; too few historians have shown such wisdom.

Some scholars have at last relinquished enough of their
ideological purity and their cherished ignorance of biology. Over the past century, a huge historical literature
has accumulated about the plague and especially the black
death, the second pandemic. At first the writing concentrated on conventional history — shifts in rulers, powers,
population, and culture. Historians argued that the black
death ended wars everywhere in Europe; enfeebled Vik-
ing settlements in Greenland and Vinland, setting back
Europe's reach toward the New World; gave rise to the
Flagellants and other heretical sects, which hastened the
splintering of Christianity; sparked bloody pogroms that
sent Jews trekking to Eastern Europe, where they developed a new culture; weakened and terrorized the Arab
world, altering its development and its relationship with
the Christian West.

As historians turned increasingly to economic theories,

they began writing about the plague's effects on trade, labor, and the distribution of wealth. By killing some of the rich and hordes of the poor, the black death helped end the feudal system. Serfs and small landowners inherited or just occupied estates whose owners had succumbed to the plague. Peasant revolts and severe labor shortages made the working class physically and economically mobile; many moved to towns, helping to form the nucleus of the urban middle class. Labor shortages and workers' new expectations may also have encouraged Europe's deep involvement in the African slave trade. Some argue (though others disagree) that reinfections and deaths were greatest in southern Europe, and that this helps to account for the northward shift of the continent's economic and cultural centers.

Several decades ago, scholars began putting the black death in a primitive biohistorical perspective. Looking at the plague as they would a big die-off in any species, they spoke of it as a curb on population growth. This view was logical but historically and biologically incomplete. Others began to look carefully at the epidemiology of the plague. They saw it as a disease of rats and their fleas, passed from rat to flea to man. It is true that the great plague pandemics were apparently brought to Europe by ship rats and then spread from ports to inland towns.

The guilty rodent in the black death was the black rat native to India, whose fleas can feed on both rats and humans. A skilled climber, it could easily scoot up mooring ropes and travel trade and exploration routes all over the world. Some historians say the black death finally faded when the black rat was ousted by the fiercer, stronger brown rat, which invaded Europe from central Asia in the early eighteenth century. The brown rat lives primarily in farmyards and sewers rather than human dwellings, and its fleas are less at home on humans than the black rat's. The black rat survived mostly as a ship rat and continued to carry the plague bacillus around the world into this century.

The idea that the plague reflected the ecological balance of man, rat, and flea is on the right track, but it doesn't explain why the plague faded when it did. The disease has kept on unaccountably hibernating and breaking out, as it did on a small scale in this country in 1983. The explanation seems to lie in a still broader view that makes the plague part of the interplay of wild rodents, rats, fleas, and changes in climate, human migration, and technology. To understand that interplay, one must look at two concepts. One is zoonoses, the diseases humans catch from other species. The other is a germ's view of survival, health, and sickness in itself and its hosts.

Yersinia pestis, the rod-shaped bacterium that causes plague, does not toil, spin, or harbor evil intent. Like any creature, it just keeps trying to survive. Bacteria are among the most ancient of living creatures, some going back perhaps two billion years. At first they probably lived in the sea and soil; then some adapted to living on and in creatures larger than themselves; some kept making further adaptations, learning to survive in still other creatures. The word zoonosis is used for a human disease caused by a germ previously at home in another species.

When a parasite moves to a new host species, it multiplies quickly, unhindered by immune reactions. It may even kill the host; then, having bitten the body that feeds it, it has no home or nourishment. If the host develops a very strong immune reaction, it can fight off or kill the parasite. The parasite's ideal relationship with its host is mutual tolerance or even symbiosis, in which each helps the other survive. This often means adapting to a particular organ or tissue. The bacteria that cause meningitis usually live peacefully in the throat; if they reach the tissue covering the brain, they become deadly. There are bacilli in the colon that graciously aid digestion; anyone who takes antibiotics is told to eat yoghurt to replace them or suffer diarrhea. If these bacilli reach the urethra and bladder, they cause stubborn, painful cystitis. Coexistence between a parasite and particular tissues takes very specialized adaptation over a long period of time.

It is therefore understandable that a germ meeting a new host takes a high death toll. For instance, when the Amerindians were first exposed to such European diseases as measles, the initial death rates were staggering. With time, the survivors and their descendants developed immune defenses; among Indians, as among Europeans, the once lethal ills became endemic — present in nearly everyone, but limited in severity. That is, they ceased to be dangerous epidemic ills of all age groups and became the less threatening ones of childhood.

A good example is the tuberculosis bacillus, perhaps one of the oldest species on earth. It had probably long been endemic in cattle when they were domesticated some ten thousand years ago. The bacillus reached humans and found it could live in them. For a long while, TB was a violent, often deadly illness, attacking almost any part of the body; a number of skeletons from ancient Egypt and Peru show severe spinal tuberculosis. With time, the germ adapted to the human lungs; then, not entirely because of antibiotics, the disease became less acute. Now healthy people all over the world who have never shown symptoms of TB show traces of immune reaction to the germ. The bacillus and humans are finally reaching a mutual adaptation that gives both a better chance to survive. Perhaps some day they will actually help each other.

Now look again at the plague. People have long noticed that the first sign of an epidemic is dead rats; apparently the plague is a new disease for them, as it is for humans. Actually, *Y. pestis* has long had a rather peaceful relationship with a variety of wild rodents, such as squirrels and voles, passed from host to host by the rodents' fleas. When black or brown rats, which are scavengers living near humans, catch the disease from wild rodents, germ and rat have both suffered a potentially dangerous accident — the classic problem of a germ passing from a familiar species to an unfamiliar one.

Biohistorian William McNeill thinks the black death began when *Y. pestis,* long endemic among wild rodents in the steppes of north and central Asia, passed to rats that had no immune defenses against it. When the rats sickened and died, the fleas and germs sought a new home in humans. The spread of the plague from central Asia may have begun partly because of stepped-up wanderings of Mongols, a result of severe climatic changes in their usual home range. Then it traveled around the world along spice-trading routes and with ship rats.

Ships rats probably continued to spread the plague into this century, passing it to wild rodents — their usual hosts — all over the world. The pandemic that struck the Pacific basin at the turn of this century left ground squirrels in California infected, and the germ spread inland from there. Public health officials think that the 1983 flare-up of the plague in the Southwest was caused by suburban expansion into areas where infected wild rodents could pass the disease to humans directly or through rats.

Some claim that with antibiotics and a reasonably good standard of living, people need no longer fear serious outbreaks of plague. Still, it remains endemic worldwide in rodents; war or disaster could tap that reservoir of infection. The plague has had a long history of killing millions and then hiding for centuries, while human immunity fades. We cannot be sure whether the disease has almost vanished or just hunkered down to wait.

It is not only trade, migrations, and shipping that have spread disease. Almost every change in our lives forces new adaptations on other species, their germs, and ours. The best example is another disease many scientists recently thought was on the way to extinction, syphilis. The history of this disease, which has become widespread again in many places, offers some of the most complicated and interesting contentions among students of human health and disease. Finally there are theories that make sense, explaining the infection as a mutual adaptation by germs to changes in human technology and life-style, and even to beliefs and attitudes.

Like typhus, syphilis exploded as a new disease in Europe in the last decade of the fifteenth century. There is a tradition that the mercenary soldiers of Charles VIII of France, who were besieging Naples, were the first to be struck by the disease. Over the next couple of years, the soldiers returned to their homes all over Europe, carrying what would soon be called the great pox (as distinguished from smallpox), a violent contagion that first showed itself with dreadful, widespread skin sores. The pox hit England in 1496, Russia in 1500; in that great age of ship exploration, it reached India in 1498, probably with Vasco Da Gama's sailors; it was carried to Canton in 1505 and Japan in 1569. Everywhere people named it for the neighboring nation that seemed to have introduced it. To the English, Germans, and Italians it was the French disease, to Frenchmen the Italian disease. Persians called it the Turkish disease. Poles called it the German disease, and Russians called it the Polish disease.

The traditional approach to the history of syphilis has been to describe the first European epidemic and name the famous rulers and artists who really or allegedly suffered the disease's late symptoms of paralysis and insanity — Charles VIII and Francis I of France, Alexander Borgia, Ivan the Terrible, perhaps Henry VIII of England, Casanova, Dürer, Cellini, Maupassant, Nietzsche. Often the list contains people such as Goya and Beethoven, to whom syphilis has been ascribed on flimsy evidence or none.

The history of syphilis is actually more complex and interesting, a bog for those who love certainty and a delight to those who like detection. The puzzle begins with the poet and physician Fracastorius, who first described typhus. In 1530, he gave the great pox its classic description in a pastoral poem called *Syphilis sive Morbus Gallicus,* "Syphilis or the French Disease," in which Syphilis, a shepherd, became the first victim of the pox as a punishment for a sin of blasphemy. (The imaginary shepherd's name would not be widely used as a name for the disease for another few centuries.) In a book on contagious diseases in 1546, Fracastorius said that the disease was often sexually transmitted and that over the past twenty years it had become less severe, its symptoms less florid.

This decreased severity has provoked one of the many contentions about the history of syphilis. One might infer that syphilis had the typical virulence of a new disease, and that after a couple of generations people began developing some defenses. Not everyone agrees. Bacteriologist Theodor Rosebury, author of an excellent history of venereal diseases, *Microbes and Morals,* doubted Fracastorius' observation. Others have pointed to a now rare form of the disease called malignant syphilis, which sometimes still occurs and has a grand, grim display of symptoms. Perhaps this was the great pox of the early sixteenth century, which subsided to the now familiar form of the disease. However, most sixteenth-century observers were convinced that syphilis was a new disease which became less violent, and this apparently also happened when the infection reached the Middle East and Asia.

If syphilis was new to Europe, where did it come from? The guess accepted until recently by most doctors and historians was that Christopher Columbus's crew or some of the Caribbean natives he brought back to Europe imported the disease from the New World. If this is true, syphilis was the only major disease that moved from the New World to the Old, rather than in the other direction.

The evidence for this idea was never solid. It first appeared a generation after the alleged event, and was popularized another generation later by a writer named Dias de Isla. Some scholars maintain that the great Fugger merchant family promoted the idea that syphilis was an American disease to boost the market for the alleged American cure they imported, guaiac wood. It did nothing for syphilis, but it did a lot for the Fuggers.

Some historians say the infection had long smoldered in Europe and for some unknown reason became fierce and epidemic in 1495. Perhaps the reason was a mutation or new strain of an old germ. There are hints of infections that might conceivably have been syphilis in ancient Hebrew, Greek, and Roman writings; perhaps syphilis was lumped together with leprosy and other disfiguring diseases from early historic times until the sixteenth century.

The clinching evidence for this theory would be bones from Europe and America, especially skulls and shin bones, which best show syphilitic damage. Throughout this century, paleopathologists have claimed to find such bones millennia old in both the New and Old Worlds, but virtually all the diagnoses are surrounded by debate. Far from all syphilitics suffer lasting bone damage, and that damage is easily confused with bone cancer, hereditary anemias, and other diseases. Leaders of each theoretical camp continue to war in specialized journals about the American or European origin of syphilis. Neither has yet convinced the other or most third parties.

Until more and better evidence turns up, this debate will remain less enlightening than a broader biohistorical view developed over several decades by Drs. Ellis Hudson, C. J. Hackett, and others. Their various versions differ in slight ways, but agree in including both the germ's view and a broad ecological and historical perspective. They see syphilis and three other diseases — pinta, yaws, and bejel — as essentially one disease, each form reflecting the germ's response to climate and to changes in human living conditions.

All four diseases are caused by a pale, corkscrew-shaped germ called a spirochete or treponeme. When the germ was isolated as the cause of syphilis early in this century, it was named *Treponema pallidum,* the pale spirochete, because it shows up white under dark-field examination through a microscope. Actually, the spirochetes that cause all four diseases cannot be distinguished under the microscope or by any laboratory test; they should probably be considered four very close strains of one species, which have evolved along with humans in a dance of mutual adaptation.

Perhaps the spirochete once lived on decaying matter, then became a parasite of primates in Africa, and some fifteen thousand years ago created a zoonosis in humans — the disease now called pinta. The spirochete's problem was its vulnerability to dryness and to extreme heat and cold; this gave it trouble surviving even briefly away from the warm moisture of the host's body. (A pre-antibiotic cure for syphilis was inducing malaria, so that the high fever would kill the spirochete and leave the patient with a manageable rather than a deadly disease.) The spirochete has had to travel quickly from one host to another, and its ways of doing so have changed along with human behavior.

Pinta is a disfiguring skin disease that now occurs in tropical areas from Mexico to Ecuador, chiefly among children, who pass it on by body contact. In a warm, wet climate, unclothed skin moistened by perspiration gives the spirochete home enough. The disease is relatively mild, not affecting the bones or internal organs. Around 10,000 B.C., says Hackett, a slight mutation in the spirochete created yaws. This, too, is transmitted among children and largely limited to the skin, but it is more severe than pinta. It became and remains common in tropical Africa.

Around 7000 B.C., when people began migrating to temperate climates and living in villages, the spirochete lost its usual home. The environment was drier and cooler, and more people's bodies were covered by clothing much of the time. The spirochete could survive only amid warmth and moisture, in the crotch, armpit, and especially the mouth. It was transmitted by kissing and common eating utensils but remained primarily a nonvenereal infection of children. The result was a new disease, bejel, also called nonvenereal or endemic syphilis. It is more severe than yaws and can attack the circulatory system and bones. It once flourished in European slums from Scotland to Russia but faded as living conditions improved. It still survives in the crowded huts of nomads, parts of northern and southern Africa, and other warm, dry regions where people usually go clothed and live in crowded village conditions. In fact, more people in the world suffer bejel than venereal syphilis.

Venereal syphilis, according to the Hudson and Hackett theories, came into existence with urban life, perhaps when the first really large cities arose in the Middle East, some six thousand years ago. In cities, people tend to live fully clothed, and the genitals become the spirochete's home, coitus the chief means of transmission, although some oral contagion remains. The disease changed its character as transmission became primarily sexual. Syphilis is mostly a disease of adults and can infect many internal organs, including the heart, bones, and central nervous system.

Ordinarily, human diseases begin as zoonoses, are acute ills of adults, and with time become less severe, the routine diseases of childhood. The pattern is oddly reversed in treponemal infections, if the Hudson-Hackett view is correct. However, there is much to support their theory. No treponemal infection exists where any other is common; each gives immunity to the others. This cross-immunity, as it is called, suggests that the germs of all four are, if not identical, very closely related. Furthermore, the change of one infection to another can be seen going on today.

When people in hot, humid lowlands suffering from yaws move to cooler mountain areas, they lose the body sores of yaws and develop those of bejel. Hudson claimed that syphilis could revert to yaws under the right climatic and living conditions. If indeed all treponemal infections are really one disease, shifting form with the climate and their hosts' way of life, such changes may have happened many times in history and are still going on. There is, in fact, a theory that the first European epidemic of syphilis was really yaws, brought to Spain from tropical Africa by slave traders; in Europe's cities and temperate climate, the germ soon ceased to cause yaws' widespread, ugly pustules and changed to syphilis — the abating severity of initial symptoms Fracastorius described.

Syphilis has continued to change recently for other reasons. In the nineteenth century, it was a devastating disease, leaving great numbers of people blind, paralyzed, and mad. The infection was often passed on by infected women (some without symptoms) to their babies in the womb; it was the source of hidden family terrors of hereditary insanity and disease. The creation of the drug Salvarsan in 1910 by Ehrlich — the first "magic bullet" of modern chemotherapy — offered some hope. The discovery of antibiotics seemed to promise unfailing cure. A few decades ago, syphilis had moved from the center of the medical curriculum to the far fringe, for eradication seemed imminent.

In the sixties, the disease started a comeback, striking teenagers and adults, afflicting male homosexuals as a silent, deadly, rectal infection. Clearly the problem was not poverty and crowding; venereal disease made its strongest revival in such prosperous nations as the United States and Sweden. Behind a facade of sexual liberation there remains a strong residue of sexual shame. This brings up one of the most intriguing aspects of the evolution of disease, the influence on it of human beliefs and attitudes — sometimes as potent as any biological force. Unfortunately, most historians, doctors, and biologists have shown utter ignorance about the sociology, psychology, and history of sex.

Venereal disease depends especially on a people's ideas, customs, and behavior. If only married couples engaged in sex, venereal disease would be virtually nonexistent. Premarital, extramarital, postmarital, and homosexual contacts are what keep it thriving. Therefore the usual

assumption is that recent sexual permissiveness lies behind
the resurgence of syphilis. However, the disease flourished
in the repressive atmosphere of the nineteenth century.
Because of guilt and secrecy, the disease was spread through
nonmarital sex, and often went untreated by terrified,
guilty victims.

Religious and social beliefs supported each other in
drawing a veil over syphilis. In 1826 Pope Leo XII banned
the condom not for preventing pregnancy but for keeping
Providence from smiting sinners where they sinned. The
attitude is not as rare today as many think, though now
people put it in nontheological but equally punitive terms:
"If people want to play around, let them take the consequences." They may or may not aid morality; they certainly help the spirochete. Politicians afraid of public
disapproval refuse to fully face the problem of venereal
disease. In Russia, China, and Cuba, where governments
fear no ballot box, syphilis has been much reduced by
rigorously tracking down the partners of each infected
person, and thus breaking the chain of infection.

It is difficult to say which has aided the spirochete more,
the guilty secrecy of puritanism or the relative relaxation
of sexual standards in recent decades. Actually, the turning point in American sex behavior came with the crucial
sexual revolution of the twenties; it may, in part, have
reflected this nation's urbanization. Kinsey's studies clearly
showed what anyone might have guessed, that city dwellers have a greater range of potential sex partners than
those in rural areas and small towns, and some take advantage of it. Syphilis, I suspect, may have been born
along with urbanization not only because of greater population density and clothing, but because of greater opportunities for venereal infection in urban people's behavior.
More syphilis can be expected as urbanization continues

all over the world. And if the trend toward divorce and remarriage continues, there will be more and more sexually active single adults, vulnerable to syphilis. Today fewer than ever use the condom, the only common contraceptive that offers significant protection against venereal infections.

The natural history of the plague and syphilis show that every aspect of human life bears in some way on health and disease, and on their impact on individuals and society. The biohistorian's approach is ecological in the truest sense, tracing the interaction of all the creatures in a changing environment. There are still other such broad approaches, which can only be suggested here. For instance, the course of human health and disease changed as our ancestors descended from the trees to the ground and adapted to a quite different ecosphere; different creatures, large and small, live in treetops than live in grass. The natural history of disease must be studied by vertical zones.

Another angle of approach is horizontal — simple population density. In cities, people create population pools that can sustain infections that would die off in smaller, thinner populations; a disease may lose its need for intermediate hosts to spread infection to humans. The growth in technology involved in urbanization also allowed people to travel all over the globe and settle in virtually every climate and environment — not only adapting to new parasites but setting off biological time bombs by upsetting old ecological balances. We have seen that even religion, attitudes, and family life affect biohistory. By comparison, the impact of drugs and vaccines may not be paramount.

Any biohistory of infectious disease must take into account the evolution of other species — parasites, hosts, and the species that affect them. We must recall that our germs and diseases didn't just leap into existence any more than we did, they evolved. Many human infections were first acquired from domesticated species, humans' scavengers, and those species' parasites. The germs of some such diseases have changed, forcing us to keep adapting to them. For instance, the influenza virus is particularly prone to mutations, and each form gives little or no immunity to the next. Flu can thus change from a temporary annoyance to a global killer of millions, as it did in the great epidemic that followed World War I — perhaps the same swine flu (again a zoonosis) many doctors feared during an aborted epidemic in 1976. Even if human flu viruses become less volatile, those from many other species would keep attacking us with dangerous force.

The smallpox virus, which has no animal reservoir, has apparently been eradicated. But the flu virus and others undergo not only mutations but frequent genetic recombinations that produce hybrids, virulent new pathogens against which we have no initial defense. New strains of the polio virus are being carried rapidly about the world by travelers, to strike unimmunized populations. Old strains of harmful viruses, long dormant, can become active again, striking populations that have lost resistance to them.

It is not only viral diseases that pose such threats. Malaria still infects some 200 million people and kills at least a million each year. In such places as Thailand and Sudan, where it was brought under control, political and economic instability have brought a resurgence. New strains of malaria parasites and of the mosquitoes that carry them have been developing resistance to chemicals that used to limit them. Furthermore, humans are just one new host for mosquitoes, which thrive on older hosts from cattle to dogs to toads. We also face an ineradicable reservoir of yellow fever in the tropical monkeys from which mosquitoes spread the disease.

The view of disease as a continuing mutual adaptation negates the notion that people once lived in a benevolent environment, a pre-urban Eden that dispensed thriving good health. It also shows that we have not emerged into a medical utopia. Man has always been a parasitologist's delight, bearing a stunning array of fungi, yeasts, protozoa, viruses, bacteria, ticks, mites, insects, and worms that seek a human host. A host is someone who prepares a table for visitors; in nature this means following the law "Eat or be eaten." Biohistorians are just starting to fully appreciate that some environments, especially warm and wet ones, present people with so many parasites to which there is no lasting immunity that world demography patterns have been strongly affected. It was such circumstances that held up for millennia the full settlement and development of vast areas of Africa and Asia.

True, many once-lethal infections are largely curable or controllable; all the world need not live in constant fear of smallpox or plague, as it has through most of history. However, new hosts and parasites keep having chance encounters that can create new diseases, even potential pestilence. Some, first seen as new diseases in a limited area, may not be quite as new or as limited as they first seem.

A good example is Lassa fever, a disease that appeared mysteriously in 1973 in Nigeria. It was eventually traced to rodents, and the high death rate among the disease's first known victims, European and American medical missionaries, suggested a new zoonosis. Now, however, researchers think the disease may have been new only to newcomers to the area. Perhaps it was long endemic in the local population, producing a quarter of a million cases of illness and tens of thousands of deaths a year, misdiagnosed as malaria or other fevers. There is still no sure answer, and no reliable treatment. So far, at least, the disease has not spread to humans and rodents about the world.

The seventies turned out to be an extraordinary decade for the appearance or first recognition of infections. Lyme disease, discovered in 1975 in Lyme, Connecticut, may be another new zoonosis. It is caused by a spirochete, transmitted by deer ticks, that is susceptible to penicillin. It hasn't proven unmanageable, though it may be more widespread than first thought.

More serious and frightening was so-called legionnaire's disease, which in 1976 struck 180 people in a Philadelphia hotel and killed twenty-nine. For six months researchers sought causes from the parrot fever germ to nickel poisoning. Finally the infection was traced to a rickettsial organism responsible for several other such outbreaks over the previous decade. Further studies showed the disease to be far from rare in New York and other big population centers; lack of recent publicity doesn't mean that the disease is a thing of the past.

That same year, a frightening and apparently new disease, viral hemorrhagic fever, killed hundreds in Zaire and Sudan. It turned out to be a variant of green monkey fever, also known as Marburg disease because it was identified in the German town of Marburg in 1967 when thirty lab technicians became sick and seven died after handling green monkeys from Uganda and Kenya. This was only one of many scares being caused by diseases reaching new parts of the world through pets and lab animals.

A rare, bizarre, but very significant disease was also explained in this period. Kuru was limited to the Fore tribe of the New Guinea highlands, where it threatened to wipe out entire villages. This infection caused degeneration of brain tissue and, invariably, death. The transmission was by ritual cannibalism; among the Fore, pregnant women and young children ate the brains of their departed, to acquire their virtues. As the practice died out, so did the disease. The importance to the rest of the world was the discovery that the cause was a slow virus.

Most viral infections incubate, erupt, and pass in days or weeks. A slow virus, such as that causing kuru, may lurk in the body for up to seven or eight years before taking effect. Such a virus causes the Creutsfeldt-Jacob syndrome, a rare and fatal form of presenile dementia with initial symptoms rather like those of Alzheimer's disease ("premature senility"). Now it is thought that slow viruses may cause such puzzling nervous-system disorders as multiple sclerosis and Parkinsonism. A clue may lie in a slow-virus disease of sheep called scrapie; perhaps we are again dealing with zoonoses.

Another possible slow-virus infection is AIDS (Acquired Immune Deficiency Syndrome), discovered in the U.S. in 1981, primarily in male homosexuals and needle-using addicts. Now this deadly disease has been found in Europe and central Africa, and in an increasing number of women and male heterosexuals. Just recently researchers in France and the U.S. have found what may be the culprit, but their research raises as many questions as it answers.

The feeling of helplessness before a deadly and uncontrollable disease is probably no different now than it was during the Great Plague. I have seen hospital staffs reduced to panic by the presence of a suspected AIDS victim. By now even a reader of these pages may be suffering a mild case of medical-student syndrome — fear of having or catching every illness whose symptoms he reads about.

Panic is out of place for most of us, but serious concern is not. As long as nature takes its familiar course, more new diseases will arise, and some old ones will become less severe. It is also true that as we keep changing our lives and our environment, we will keep creating risks that will challenge medical ingenuity to its utmost. Human migrations are bigger and faster than ever in history. Parasites and their carriers are moving about the world at a dizzy ecological pace; they are also evolving rapidly in response to pesticides and drugs. The arrival, change, and subsidance of diseases are part of an ancient balancing act, but they have speeded up to a frenetic pace, without the time for gradual adaptations that used to exist. As we better understand the dance of health and disease in the past and present, we see incalculable changes ahead. And as the following chapter shows, we must even face risks to the entire biosphere, not from germs but from the contents of the earth itself.

7

Global Poison

THE AILING BIOSPHERE

We have seen how the changing forces of nature and of illness shape the lives of individuals, societies, the entire world. There is another form of biocataclysm, and it may soon visit us as the disease that changed Goya's life. Once lead poisoning was probably only the malady of certain occupations, though some surmise that it has undermined empires. In recent decades it has especially endangered young children around the world, especially in cities. Tomorrow lead poisoning may afflict the entire human species. This subtle, versatile poison is piling up in our air and water, our crops and animals, our very bones.

Recent reliance on iron and steel can make us forget how vital lead has always been to technological man. In fact, it has probably been written about more through history than any other toxic agent; the study of lead poisoning is a major source of industrial medicine, industrial-hygiene legislation, and toxicology. Lead was one of the first metals used by man, for its low melting point and malleability make it easy to smelt and shape. The Egyptians used lead more than five thousand years ago; the British Museum possesses a lead statuete from the First

Dynasty. They also used it for dishes, rings, amulets, sinkers for fishing nets, and pigment in eye paint. Other peoples of the eastern Mediterranean mined and worked lead; the tribute lists of Pharaoh Thutmosis III (circa 1500 B.C.) show that his armies brought it home as spoils from Mesopotamia. Lead was used from kitchens to shipyards and, because of its softness, could serve as either pencil or slate. Many ancient slates have survived, especially "curse slates" smuggled into enemies' graves to invite nastiness from demons and evil spirits.

Lead was also used in ancient India, for amulets and loom weights, and in China and pre-Columbian Mexico. The Old Testament mentions the metal. Large amounts first became available as a byproduct of cupellation, a process for separating out the silver that often lies in lead-rich ore. Cupellation was probably discovered by tribes on the coast of the Black Sea some forty-five hundred years ago and then spread. It is mentioned in the Book of Jeremiah, and through its use Athens drew much of its silver wealth from the famous Laurion mines.

Expanding Greco-Roman technology demanded more and more lead: for reinforcement in construction; for hoops and bands, where now we use steel wire; for anchors, battering rams, and sling shots; for coins; for household utensils; for vessels to store water and oil. It protected ship bottoms from worms; a recently salvaged Greek wine ship built around 150 B.C. bore two hundred tons of cast-lead sheathing. Reservoirs, aqueducts, and water mains were lined with lead from Rome to the Rhône valley. It was also made into pipes and plummets — hence our words plumbing and plumb bob, from *plumbus,* the Latin word for lead. Roman wrestlers fastened bits of lead to the leather thongs they wrapped about their hands and arms. The women of Athens and Rome used white oxide of lead as a cosmetic. Minium, the red oxide of lead, was used to color and flavor wine, which was stored in lead vats.

It is no surprise, then, to find lead poisoning in the earliest annals of medicine. Hippocrates noted that miners suffered from pallor, tense abdomen, and enlargement of the spleen; when a convict was sentenced to work in the mines, it was a sentence to death. The poet and physician Nicander, in the second century B.C., described plumbism in detail. Pliny mentioned the ravages of lead, mercury, and sulphur, and the poisoning caused by lead in pottery glazes, food additives, and storage vessels. Refiners of minium, he said, tried to protect themselves by using animal bladders as face masks — one of the first attempts at industrial hygiene on record.

The hazards of mining and working with metals were obviously common knowledge; they were noted by Martial, Juvenal, and Lucretius. Vitruvius, in the first great treatise in architecture, warned that water conducted in lead pipes is less healthful than that in pipes of clay, "because lead is found to be harmful. . . . This we can exemplify from plumbers, since in them the natural color of the body is replaced by a deep pallor." The emperor Augustus forbade the use of lead pipes for potable water, but his decree, like so many attempts through history to limit people's exposure to lead, was probably enforced spottily.

The production of lead fell with Roman civilization. Then records of lead mining reappear around the tenth century, in eastern Germany. As farming and barter gave way to industry, trade, and money, the demand for metals soared. Lead was needed for all the old uses and new ones as well, from firearms shot to printers' type. Deep mining developed, and producing iron, gold, silver, and lead became major industries. Once again people began to fear metals' effects. In the 1470s Ulrich Ellenbog, a physician in Augsburg, wrote a treatise on the ills of workers in gold, mercury, and lead; it circulated in manuscript form and was finally printed in the early 1520s.

In 1567 the first work was written devoted entirely to the ills of miners, smelters, and metal workers — *On the Miners' Sickness and Other Diseases of Miners*. The author bore the glorious name Theophrastus Bombastus von Hohenheim, which he gave up to become known as Paracelsus. This cantankerous Swiss-born physician, chemist, alchemist, and student of the occult was ousted from university after university for both his irascibility and his innovative ideas. In his own premature, one-man scientific revolution, he dismissed the humoral theory of disease and stressed clinical observation and specific remedies. Unfortunately, he also made claims for the medicinal properties of opium, mercury, and lead.

During the sixteenth century more works on mining and its hazards appeared; authors also began discussing the health of soldiers, seafarers, salt workers, scholars. Still, no one conceived of occupational ills as a distinct branch of medicine till almost 1700 when Bernardino Ramazzini, a doctor in the Italian city of Modena, achieved scientific greatness as many others have, by stopping to question the ordinary. In this case, the ordinary was the cleaning of sewers. Ramazzini described the golden, malodorous moment (I condense):

"At this point I invite doctors to leave the apothecary's shop, redolent of cinnamon, and come to the latrines. In this city it is the custom to clean each house's sewers every three years. While this was going on at my house, I watched the workman and saw that he looked very apprehensive and was straining every nerve. I pitied him at that filthy work and asked him why he was working so strenuously and did not take it more quietly, to avoid overexertion. The poor wretch lifted his eyes from the cavern, gazed at me, and said: 'No one who has not tried it can imagine what it costs to stay more than four hours in this place; it is the same thing as being struck blind.' "

Ramazzini examined the man's eyes and found them badly bloodshot. Did privy cleaners have a remedy? Only, he learned, to shut themselves in the dark and bathe their eyes with lukewarm water to relieve the pain a bit. "After that," wrote Ramazzini, "I saw several workers of this class with eyes half-blinded or stone-blind begging for alms in the town. . . . I am inclined to think that some volatile acid is given off by this camerine of filth when they disturb it."

There most people would stop, but for Ramazzini the observation was a beginning. He was not only a charming man, with the true healer's human concern, but a pragmatic citizen who knew health's importance for society's well-being and prosperity. And he had the innovator's relentless curiosity and intolerance for facts without contexts. For years he haunted Modena's workshops, examining and questioning. In 1700 his *Discourse on the Diseases of Workers* appeared, describing the ills of forty-two occupational groups from gilders, painters, and potters to singers and midwives. An expanded edition of 1713 contained a dozen new chapters on such workers as printers, weavers, well-diggers, and scholars.

The first chapter of this founding classic of occupational medicine dealt with miners, and Ramazzini singled out lead for its destructiveness — a cause of "dyspnoea, phthisis, apoplexy, paralysis, cachexia, swollen feet, loss of teeth, ulcerated gums, pains in the joints and palsy." Lead hangs heavy over much of the book. In the chapter on potters, Ramazzini describes visiting and revisiting their workshops, seeking the cause of their notoriously poor health. He found it in their lead glazes. The symptoms of lead miners and potters reappeared in the chapter on painters, along with plumbism's melancholia.* The source was lead and mercury pigments.

Ramazzini passed on a few traditional remedies, with more hope than confidence. Imperiled craftsmen should quit their trades; in reality, too many were chained to their jobs by poverty or lack of other opportunities. By the time they sought help, many were already beyond the mercies of treatment or time. Potters went to doctors only when "their feet and hands are totally crippled and their internal organs have become very hard; and they suffer from yet another drawback, I mean that they are very poor." Then, as today, there was second-class medicine for second-class citizens. Finally, Ramazzini had to quote Hippocrates: "We must study incurable ailments so that they may hurt the patient as little as possible."

A small touch of hope lay in prevention. Mines should be ventilated, the workers given gloves and leggings. Many arsenic workers wore glass masks; minium polishers should imitate those described by Pliny, who tied bladders over their faces to avoid inhaling noxious dust.

This still amounted to little real help. Ramazzini's gift to medicine was not marvelous new therapies but a new concept. Hippocrates, he said, had listed what a doctor should learn when he first visits a patient — what sort of

---

*Ramazzini did allow that painters' "sedentary life and melancholic temperament may also be partly to blame, for they are almost entirely cut off from intercourse with other men and constantly absorbed in the creations of their imagination." Ramazzini's last word was typically pragmatic. As a case of the mind disordered by lead he gave Correggio, who "is said to have been so melancholic, not to say stupid, that he failed to realize his own pre-eminence and the value of his paintings, so much so that he would pay back his well-earned fees to those from whom he had received them. . . ."

pains he has, what caused them, how long he has been sick, his diet, and the workings of his bowels. "I may venture," said Ramazzini, "to add one more question: What occupation does he follow?"

The century following Ramazzini's book saw few major advances in occupational medicine or in understanding plumbism. The illness kept being ignored and rediscovered through recent years. For instance, doctors have regularly stumbled over the dangers of improperly glazed pottery, and of acid substances activating the lead in glaze or alloy. Lead peweter caused lead colic in the American colonies, and in 1723 the Massachusetts Bay Colony outlawed the making of rum in leaded stills to prevent "dry gripes" — lead colic. This was the first industrial hygiene legislation in the American colonies. Three decades later in England, James Lind, who had discovered that citrus fruits prevent scurvy, warned against storing acidic fruit juice in earthenware jugs. In 1767 Sir George Baker blamed the endemic colic of Devonshire on apple cider stored in lead-lined troughs and mentioned similar past endemics in Europe. Ben Franklin noted that people in many trades, including his own occupation of printing, were susceptible to lead poisoning.

Two centuries later similar cases were still cropping up. In 1970 researchers at McGill University reported that two children's lead poisoning had been traced to apple juice their mother kept in an earthenware jug, and a physician's plumbism to drinking cola beverage from a glazed mug made by his son. The McGill scientists tested almost 170 earthenware food and beverage containers and common glazes; excessive lead was leached from almost half of them. Hundreds of millions of drinking glasses with lead-bearing decorations were made in the U.S. in 1977, and millions were then taken off the market. The Colonial rum makers also have twentieth-century counterparts. Many moonshiners use old automobile radiators as condensers in their stills; some, like brewers of antiquity and the Middle Ages, even add lead — now in the form of battery plates — to improve the flavor. Saturnine gout and the lead encephalopathy from which Goya suffered have often been traced to lead-contaminated mountain dew.

Such cases are, unfortunately, but a small fraction of lead poisoning's toll since the industrial revolution. The nineteenth century's terrible mines, mills, and slums imposed squalid urban serfdom on millions. This new tide of poverty and illness demanded remedies, and they began arriving as labor regulations, public-health measures, and industrial hygiene. At the same time, progress in medicine and chemistry speeded research on occupational disease. Plumbism's colic, palsy, and death were widespread enough to draw intense interest.

In 1839 Tanquerel des Planches described lead encephalopathy and noted plumbism's telltale blue line on the gums, caused by lead deposits. By midcentury, physicians had learned that lead can cause miscarriage and stillbirth; many women already knew that and used lead to induce abortion, and sometimes suffered acute lead poisoning as a result. By the 1880s a clear clinical picture of plumbism had developed, and research in England, Germany, and the U.S. went on to show how lead affects the body. It causes anemia by interfering with red blood cells; damages the kidneys, sometimes permanently, and leaves chemical clues in the urine; produces degeneration in nerve cells that results in palsy and crippling; crosses the placenta and poisons infants in the womb; alters sperm cells so that a man's plumbism may fatally deform his offspring. By 1926 J. C. Aub and his colleagues knew enough to write the first major book on lead poisoning, bringing together a wide range of medical, chemical, and industrial knowledge.

By now lead's worst industrial ravages were being eliminated or reduced, and the metal was disappearing from many common products. Far less frequently did doctors see the convulsions, blindness, and hallucinations of acute lead encephalopathy; earlier, milder symptoms were more often detected and treated. Lead poisoning was at last considered a rare and usually minor disease. Research began slowing to a trickle of studies on lead's complex effects on body chemistry and cell functions. The relief was premature.

Little outbreaks kept occurring. Some were caused by lead-lined beer vats; by fumes from the burning of old auto batteries; by scraping and painting, as in the bridge painters of Dusseldorf described in chapter two; perhaps by tobacco plant pesticide containing lead arsenate. Physicians themselves gave lead anemia a brief comeback in the late 1920s, when intravenous lead injections had a vogue in cancer treatment. There is a story that during World War II, glassmakers in occupied Czechoslovakia deliberately increased the lead in glass made for export to Germany. An unexpected case arose in April 1974, when the Health Research Group associated with Ralph Nader insisted that the government ban candlewicks stiffened with lead. These burning wicks, they claimed, released enough lead fumes to constitute a health hazard.

Alarm over leaded candlewicks may suggest that plumbism is now an exotic malady. But that same month, another outbreak of plumbism occurred that opens the door on a frightening new dimension of the illness. The victims were demolition workers dismantling the tracks of the old

Third Avenue El in the Bronx, and the case evokes Pliny, Ramazzini, and all the others through history who have repeated the ancient knowledge that lead is a poison.

A crew of twelve "precutters" had the task of burning most of the way through heavy metal beams before they were cut loose and removed by a crane. The cutting torches vaporized not only metal but an eighty-three-year accumulation of lead-base paint. The men wore respirators, but fortunately that wasn't reassurance enough for some doctors who read about the job and recalled outbreaks of lead poisoning during previous El demolitions. An occupational-health team from the Environmental Sciences Laboratory of Mount Sinai Medical Center and members of the City Health Department visited the site. They tested the precutters' blood for lead and found no reason for concern. But another check six weeks later revealed a steep rise in blood lead levels, and a third test soon afterward showed dangerous amounts. A few men reported cramps and constipation — lead colic. At this rate, many would soon suffer serious, even lethal, damage to their kidneys and brains.

The precutters began going each morning to Mount Sinai Hospital, where calcium EDTA was dripped into their veins. This chemical clasps lead in the blood in a stable chemical bond; the kidneys then safely filter it out and excrete it.

The vigilant health team located the reason for the poisoning. Each man's respirator shquld have been supplied by its own air pump. Instead, two or three respirators were linked by hoses to a single pump. Inadequate air pressure beneath the face masks sucked in outside air, and with it lead fumes. Sometimes the precutters worked utterly unprotected. One worker said, "Sometimes we wouldn't get enough air and the masks would tighten up on our faces, and we would have to take them off." The head of the demolition company told *The New York Times,* "We've demolished half a dozen Els using the same equipment and never had the problem before." He also admitted there had been no blood tests before.

Such old paint as sickened the precutters has made lead poisoning a mass crippler and killer of children. Dangerous lead pigment was widely replaced in paint in the U.S. around 1940 by nontoxic titanium dioxide, but its presence on old dilapidated houses is a lingering hazard to the young, especially those with a peculiar behavior called pica.

Pica is Latin for magpie, a bird of voracious and varied appetite; it means habitually eating things usually considered nonfoods, such as clay, laundry starch, paper, and, very commonly, paint chips. Pica has been known since antiquity and occurs all around the world, yet it remains poorly understood. During children's first year of life, they mouth almost anything, but without necessarily swallowing. Then between twelve and eighteen months, many start eating nonfoods. The behavior fades out between ages three and five except in a small minority; prolonged pica may be caused by brain damage — sometimes the result of lead poisoning.

Decades ago, doctors thought pica a signal of diet deficiency, but now we know that many children with pica are well nourished. Furthermore, pica is not limited to children; it occurs in adults, especially pregnant women. In fact, the mother-child relationship may be crucial in pica; in some studies as many as half the mothers of pica children show pica themselves. At all ages, chewing and eating can reflect or reduce anxiety, as every compulsive nibbler knows. A poor, overworked mother swamped by responsibilities may exhibit pica. So may a child under stress; pica sometimes appears when a sibling arrives or when the mother is overwhelmed by problems.

Pica may also have a cultural source. Clay-eating is a common habit among blacks in some parts of the rural South. Anxious, burdened mothers there may give distressed toddlers the clay or laundry starch they themselves chew, as a substitute for a bottle or pacifier. Some researchers say that many rural Southern blacks take the pica habit to Northern cities and lose it after several generations, especially after winning greater economic and social security. That many people with pica prefer one or two substances certainly suggests cultural influence rather than indiscriminate oral or dietary needs.

A still more recent theory says that pica is not a disorder but a normal phase of development. It has been seen in up to 50 percent of children, in middle-class homes as well as slums and poor farm country. It is too early to confidently label pica normal or an anxiety behavior reinforced by tradition. Whatever the behavior's nature, a pica-prone toddler in a dilapidated house with cracked, peeling paint faces the worst ravages of lead poisoning.

Pica was first related to lead poisoning some fifty years ago, but only in the past few decades has the problem been recognized as a lethal endemic. In the early 1950s most major cities reported only a few cases of plumbism a year. Slowly awareness grew, and city after city roused itself enough to carry out screening programs, especially in slums. Hundreds of cases appeared, then thousands. Some seven hundred were reported in New York City in 1968; in 1970 the figure rose to about twenty-five hundred. Using complex methods of analyzing urine, feces, or blood, researchers carried out surveys in large and middle-sized cities across the country. The results were sadly similar in old neighborhoods of Chicago, Baltimore, New Haven, Norfolk, and Washington: some 5 to 10 percent of children showed high lead levels, and 1 to 2 percent suffered undiagnosed lead poisoning. In the worst slums, an estimated 10 to 25 percent of children were taking in too much lead, and 2 to 5 percent needed treatment. A screening of a half million children in sixty cities in the late seventies showed high lead levels in about 5 percent. Lead was not only a problem of the poor; it was increasing in children of the affluent who rehabilitated old inner-city dwellings.

Multiplying these results to a national level shows that lead poisoning may be the single worst threat to American children's life and health, far outstripping the dangers of the most feared infectious diseases. This is no surprise if one remembers how dense the lead becomes on a heavily repainted wall, porch, or pipe. A paint chip the size of an adult's thumbnail may contain a hundred milligrams of lead. The adult body excretes only half of one milligram a day and retains the rest. So one old, dense chip may hold one or two hundred times the "safe" adult intake; a few small chips a day can transmit more lead than a heavily exposed industrial worker receives. Children's digestive systems may absorb a far greater percent of ingested lead than adults'. And they are far more vulnerable to lead's ravages, especially in their immature nervous systems.

Parents and doctor confronted by a crying twenty-month-old will be baffled by plumbism's lack of distinctive symptoms. What should they make of various degrees and combinations of fatigue, lack of appetite, constipation, vomiting, irritability, headache, bellyache, and anemia? As they ponder myriad disorders, the child may go on to stupor, coma, and convulsions; these could signal meningitis or brain tumor. Everything depends on the parents' and doctor's awareness of plumbism as a possibility. Lead-poisoned children, like adults, can be treated with chelating substances; *chēlē* is Greek for claw, and its English derivative denotes molecules that grasp metal atoms firmly in soluble form. Calcium EDTA can clear a great deal of lead from the body, but it cannot reverse much of the damage done to the kidneys and brain.

Even a decade ago, some optimists thought that only about two hundred children died each year in the U.S. of plumbism, a figure that put the disease among medical exotica. But that figure was probably low considering how many cases are undiscovered and misdiagnosed. In some recently treated groups of severely poisoned children, the death rate has been as low as 5 percent, but the aftereffects of encephalopathy crippled from one-quarter to three-quarters of the survivors. Those who are reexposed to lead almost invariably suffer permanent damage. At least six hundred thousand children are poisoned to some degree by lead each year, and we should not watch only those left with cerebral palsy, blindness, epilepsy, or severe mental retardation. Many more suffer in previously undetected ways.

As people recognized that plumbism is a plague, research centered on the silent epidemic of subtle deficits in learning and behavior. It is insidious and frightening because it appears in many children who show high blood lead if tested but never exhibit the symptoms of poisoning. Asymptomatic high blood lead is responsible for many children being labeled retarded, slow learner, or hyperactive. Other effects are even more subtle, and only a little less damaging. A New Haven study of symptom-free, lead-exposed children revealed fine-motor and language problems. Drs. Julian Chisholm, Jr., and Eugene Kaplan found that even lead-exposed children with good school records and high IQ scores may have mild distortions in visual perception, tending to break down a drawing into its components rather than seeing it as a whole. They may also show what Chisholm and Kaplan call perseveration:

"For example, if you teach the child that 5 × 5 is 25 and then ask him what 4 × 3 is, the child says 25. . . . Once he learns a correct answer, he repeats it even when the question is changed. The unwitting teacher (or mother) may conclude that such a child is insolent, whereupon she will punish him and so reinforce and aggravate the behavioral problems often present in such children . . . many lead-poisoned children develop hostile, aggressive and destructive behavior patterns."

Brain damage is lead poisoning's most dramatic sequel, but not the only one. Back in the 1920s, in Australia, kidney damage was linked to widespread plumbism caused by drinking rainwater collected on roofs coated with lead-base paint. In 1954 a follow-up study tracked down about three hundred fifty adults who had been lead-poisoned fifteen to forty years earlier. Almost half were already dead, nearly a hundred from kidney disease. An American study a decade later had less dramatic results, but it does seem that early lead poisoning can create lasting or progressive kidney damage.

Research continues on how lead acts in the body, and it suggests a more complex picture than early investigators could have imagined. The lead we can't excrete must find storage sites, and lead is a bone-seeker; 90 percent of the body's stored lead is normally in the skeleton, where it displaces calcium. There it rests in a stable reservoir until it reaches some threshold, different for each person and different over time for each individual. Then a little more lead or any trauma — a fracture, fever, changes in body chemistry — may make the bones dump lead back into the bloodstream. That is why, in some cases, lead accumulates in lethal amounts without causing symptoms, and then suddenly acute poisoning appears.

Some of this circulating lead enters red blood cells, interfering with hemoglobin synthesis and causing anemia. The rest prefers certain soft tissues: hair, where it is harmless; the liver, which functions despite moderate amounts; the kidneys, which suffer moderate to severe damage; the brain and peripheral nerves; the thyroid, where iodine uptake is slowed; the aorta, which shows pathological changes; other blood vessels and the heart. And as we noted, lead can deform or kill the fetus by affecting sperm cells or passing through the placenta to the embryo's blood, bones, and soft tissues. It can even reach an infant through the mother's milk.

Many conditions and substances can increase one's vulnerability to lead and trigger or heighten its effects. Some people may have a genetic susceptibility. Alcoholism, kidney disease, and anemia raise the risk. Among the physiological triggers is sunlight. Pica victims consume lead all year, but 85 percent of acute poisonings appear from May through October. Probably summer sunlight stimulates the creation of vitamin D, which in turn raises lead absorption in the intestine. Another trigger is a deficiency of chromium, a trace metal we need in small amounts. Chromium deficiency afflicts not only the underfed but many overweight, affluent eaters of junk snacks and overprocessed foods. Besides producing its own symptoms, chromium deficiency increases the effects of lead. Further, when lead is fed to chromium-deficient rats, they catch more infections and have a much lower survival rate; the low-chromium/high-lead combination seems to suppress the body's powers of immuniy. Deficiencies in phosphate, iron, protein, vitamins C and D, nicotinic acid, and several other substances have been similarly implicated.

A particularly interesting suspicious bystander is calcium. Lead easily replaces it not only in the bones but in the environment. Some water may even be "soft" — that is, low in calcium — because environmental lead has replaced the element that once made it hard. The results have long been known: back around the turn of this century, the very low birth rate in Dewsbury, England, was traced to the high lead content of the local water. If lead is, in fact, replacing calcium in water supplies, it may be having subtle effects on the birth, life, and death of large populations. It would also be logical to assume that lead has done so in the past. There is even a theory that lead poisoning helped topple the Roman empire.

This idea, interesting in itself and for its modern implications, saw print as early as 1824, when A. Henderson, in a history of wines, pointed out the very large amount of lead in Roman food and drink. In the 1880s a few German and Austrian toxicologists pursued the question. First they found hundreds of bits of evidence in ancient writings. Then, seeking physical evidence, they studied the bones of several dozen ancient Romans and found lead. They fell short of proving a saturnine plague in antiquity because chemical methods then could reveal only the presence of lead in bones, not its exact amount. Their findings lay almost ignored until S. C. Gilfillan, a California scientist, took up the idea again in the early 1960s.

Gilfillan's argument, in brief, is this. Roman culture started to decline in the second or first century B.C., partly because the upper class began rapidly dying out, and with them much of the empire's educated, creative leadership — at precisely the time when the introduction of Greek cookery brought lead poisoning to the affluent. Greece itself had undergone a similar decline a few centuries earlier. The less wealthy of Rome and Greece consumed far less lead, so they did not suffer plumbism's lower birthrate, increased child mortality, and mental impairment.

Much of Rome's water-supply system was made of lead; the Greeks collected rainwater from lead-lined roofs and stored oil in lead-lined vessels. The Greeks also used lead widely in food and wine; in this, as in many other things, the Romans followed them to excess. The Romans used lead in their wine in at least fourteen ways, such as heating wine in lead vessels and sweetening it with grape syrup boiled long, with much scraping, in lead pots. They used the same lead-impregnated grape syrup to preserve foods. Honey cooked in lead was a common laxative. We have already seen that Vitruvius, Galen, and Pliny noted the ill effects of lead on food and water; Greek writers also observed that certain wines produced sterility, miscarriage, constipation, headache — all symptoms of plumbism. And lead, we noted, was a common cosmetic and industrial metal. Many Romans of the first two centuries of this era may have used almost as much lead as Americans do today — two or more pounds per person each year.

Gilfillan, unlike his precessors in the biohistory of lead, had methods for measuring the amount of lead in ancient bones. He had analyses made of bones from forty Greeks and Romans of the suspect period; the lead content, as he had predicted, was high. He also studied estimates of birth and death rates and concluded that the Roman upper class did dwindle dramatically for six centuries after the importation of Greece's lead-laden culinary luxuries, around 150 B.C.

Gilfillan's essay leaves many doubts. Some of his assertions about both plumbism and history seem sweeping and liable to other explanations; some even beg argument. Gilfillan himself points out that the fall of Rome has been a favorite subject "for every curbstone amateur, and that each tends to ascribe that downfall to whatever evil most oppose today." Historians have blamed bloated government bureaucracy, economic and population pressures, slavery, malaria, plague, soil exhaustion, and tribes pushed from central Asia by climatic change. A true answer, Gilfillan admits, must include them all. But his favorite culprit, despite soft spots in his argument, sticks in one's mind. His theory was amplified in 1983 in *The New England Journal of Medicine* by Dr. Jerome Nriagu of Canada.

Nriagu covers much the same ground as Gilfillan, with the same overtone of moralism, but he emphasizes another point — the relationship between a rich, lead-laced diet and gout. Gout, he claims, was common in the overprivileged and overfed of Rome. Art and writings also suggest a virtual epidemic of gout among affluent feasters and topers of eighteenth-century England. They, like the Romans, consumed lots of wine fortified with lead; much of their food and drink was stored, prepared, and served in lead-bearing utensils.

Nriagu, like Gilfillan, sometimes begs argument. If saturnine gout so ravaged eighteenth-century Britons, why didn't their empire crumble the same way, with the same demographic disaster? Furthermore, paleopathologists have argued convincingly that gout was not common but rare in ancient Rome. At most, we can accept lead as one possible factor among many in the fall of empires. Perhaps the Gilfillan and Nriagu theories have won some popularity because lead is now so pervasive in our environment that some researchers fear subclinical lead poisoning has become a silent threat to the entire world.

The bones of prehistoric man contain virtually no lead, and the metal isn't needed for life or health. Very simply, lead entered man's body when he began to use it. In 1838 French scientists Devergie and Hervy were the first to suggest an idea which would long be argued — that lead is normally present in man. Unfortunately, in technological man it is true. Yet there has not been the same loud, public crusade against lead as against DDT and carbon monoxide, though in the long run it may be more dangerous. DDT and carbon monoxide eventually break down to harmless components, but lead, a relatively inert element, never becomes biodegradable. Once it enters the biosphere, much of it is likely to stay there, cycling and recycling through rain, snow, crops, animals, and man.

A dramatic example of lead's course through the environment to man occurred in the Belgian town of Hoboken in 1974. A woman who lived near there took some of her hay to her sister-in-law's farm, six miles away. The cows ate the hay and died a few weeks later; a veterinarian's postmortem verdict was lead poisoning. The news spread back to Hoboken and made farmers there think of recent disturbing events on their property — leaves falling inexplicably from the trees on a sunny day, poultry dying mysteriously, horses and cows dropping dead in the fields. It took no detective to find the source. In Hoboken stood a plant that refined 25,000 tons of lead a year, dispensing lead dust and fumes from its smokestacks and slagheaps.

Health officials warned people in and around Hoboken not to eat vegetables from their gardens. But people there were less concerned about the vegetables than about their children, so the nation's Ministry of Health tested fifty local youngsters of ages five and six. Then they refused to release the results, even to the parents and to local authorities.

The company promptly paid reparations for dead livestock and started taking expensive measures to reduce the pollution. Interestingly, its spokesman said the processes used there were the same ones used seventy-five years earlier, when the plant opened; pollution may have been no worse than before, but people were more aware and frightened. The plant went on operating without massive opposition, for it provided Hoboken with 2,500 jobs and $175,000 a year in taxes. A similar situation came to light in the El Paso area. A century-old smelter was shown to have raised the body lead of ten thousand or more children; it may well have damaged the brain function of hundreds or thousands.

These are not isolated incidents. A study in Ireland showed that almost 2 percent of the cattle tested and 4.5 percent of the calves suffered from lead poisoning. Horses have died of lead-contaminated hay not only in Belgium but in England and California; near some smelters, horses cannot be raised at all. Ewes in high-lead areas suffer frequent abortions. In fact, several researchers have said that lead is now the commonest poisoner of domesticated animals, and some of that lead enters our food chain.

Oysters and clams have a strong affinity for lead; some in lead-contaminated waters of the Atlantic and Gulf Coast could cause plumbism if eaten in large amounts. Many wildfowl also contain too much lead; the cause is not smelters but ammunition. "Fill him with lead" and "he died of lead poisoning" aren't mere figures of speech. Many people who carry metal fragments from gunshot wounds suffer severe or even fatal lead poisoning. Lead shot is now commonest in bird-hunters' shotguns; at least six thousand tons of it are expended in this country each year. Some lakes along bird-migration paths have been shot over so much that the bottoms are blanketed with lead pellets. Birds, lacking teeth, swallow gravel to grind the food in their crops; wild waterfowl now swallow so much lead in gravel from lakes and streams that 2 to 3 percent (about a million birds a year) die of lead poisoning — among them such endangered species as bald eagles and whooping cranes. Doubtless many more birds fail to breed. Some of the lead in birds directly or indirectly enters our food chain and water supply.

In the U.S., less lead has been used over the past half-century in paint and consumer products, but the reduction has easily been equaled by the use of lead tetraethyl (TEL), an antiknock gasoline additive expelled from the exhaust pipes of motor vehicles. TEL constitutes half the lead absorbed by city dwellers. In the country, airborne lead falls on vegetation, soil, and water. Grass and weeds near a well-traveled road can contain enough lead to cause abortion or even overt plumbism in a cow that eats them exclusively. The lead can also reach us through vegetables growing near highways. Dr. Henry A. Schroeder, perhaps the world's leading authority on the effects of trace metals, has tested melted snow from such an area. Of twenty samples, fifteen held more lead than the legal safety limit for drinking water; seven samples contained five times that limit.

But the worst threat from airborne lead is direct inhalation. We have seen that the adult body retains 10 percent of the lead we swallow, but a much higher proportion of the lead we inhale. The amount depends on the size and solubility of the particles; estimates for TEL have varied from less than 20 percent to 50 percent or even more, but 35 to 45 percent may be a good guess. The chemical form of this lead is especially unfortunate. In organic (synthetic) compounds, many metals become more toxic; when lead is combined with ethyl groups, it may be very toxic indeed, with more propensity for brain and liver cells than for bone. So inhaling TEL probably does far more damage than swallowing an equal amount of inorganic lead compounds.

TEL was first added to gasoline in the U.S. in 1924 with knowledge that it might be dangerous. The U.S. Public Health Service (PHS) held conferences about it in 1925 and 1926 and concluded that existing evidence did not justify banning it. A small number of poisonings, deaths, and severe psychiatric disorders were traced to TEL as decades passed, but the lack of lead-poisoned bodies strewn about the nation apparently stilled apprehensions. More TEL entered the world's atmosphere from 1940 on, as many other nations started using TEL and more vehicles came into use.

In 1965 the PHS reexamined TEL, but there was little new knowledge; the government had sponsored almost no research on it. What new data existed came largely from studies financed by General Motors and Dupont, the major TEL manufacturers. A 1961–62 survey in Cincinnati, Philadelphia, and Los Angeles had revealed no plumbism caused by TEL, so again it was not banned or limited. But this time there was dissent, and some of it sounded caustic.

Dr. Harry Heimann of the Harvard School of Public Health sarcastically pointed out the lack of evidence that "a little lead is good for you." After talk about lead-tolerance levels, an HEW official stated flatly, "Lead is not tolerable." Eminent lead researcher Clair C. Patterson, a geochemist at the California Institute of Technology, criticized the PHS for setting permissible lead levels too high. John C. Esposito, a consumer advocate writing on air pollution, called federal inaction a whitewash based on industry-financed research: "For researchers concerned with atmospheric lead to look almost exclusively for symptoms as acute as [overt plumbism] is absurd; it is as if carbon monoxide researchers were looking only for asphyxiation."

Memories of some research claims by the tobacco and drug industries, among others, justify suspicion. It isn't reassuring to note the downplaying of danger and resistance to lowering legal lead thresholds by the lead, oil, and auto industries. Nevertheless, large corporations do often finance skilled and honest researchers, and some of those who saw no lead terror in the air are widely respected for their work on lead physiology. Outrage and paranoia take one no closer to the truth than corporate fact-bending, and finally health legislation must be based on strong evidence and sound interpretation. We can learn a great deal about environmental lead by testing the air, rain, snow, and the lead-bearing dust that pollutes them.

Street dust in many American cities shows increased lead since TEL went into use. A 1971 study of snow collected within one hundred feet of streets and roads in Columbus, Ohio, revealed that seventeen of twenty-seven samples exceed PHS safety limits for lead in drinking water. Lead is found increasingly in our oceans, especially off industrial coasts. The lead in water and air, we know, enters vegetation; Swedish research has shown excessive lead in mosses and tree rings, in patterns corresponding with the use of industrial lead and leaded gas. But the best measure of lead pollution probably lies in Arctic glaciers; much volatile lead eventually reaches the upper atmosphere and is deposited there in snow. Measurements near the poles aren't affected by local factories, winds, and other special influences.

Clair Patterson published in 1969 a study of lead in

glacial ice from northern Greenland. The ice showed little lead till about the ninth century, but the amount increased tenfold from the tenth to eighteenth centuries; in 1753, around the start of Europe's industrial revolution, it had reached twenty-five times the natural (pretechnological) level. Lead tripled during the period 1753 1815, doubled again in 1815–1933, and tripled once more in 1933–1965. By 1965 lead was well over five hundred times the natural level. The sharpest rise had started around 1940, as a result of lead alkyls.

A very direct test of how lead in all its forms has encroached on us is that used to study plumbism in antiquity — measuring the lead in bones, where it accumulates as a person ages. Studies of bones from third-century Poland and from a Peruvian mummy buried around A.D. 1200 reveal little or no lead. Bones from eleventh-century Europe contain a rather large amount, presumably from pewter and lead utensils. (A notable case of medieval plumbism appeared in 1959, when the body of Clement VII, who held the papacy in 1046–1047, was removed from its stone coffin in Bamberg; so much lead was found in one of his ribs that researchers concluded he had died of lead poisoning.) In the Middle Ages, probably only lead workers, residents near smelters, and the affluent were highly exposed; lead had not yet suffused the world's air and water. But in the 1950s, Henry Schroeder compared bone and tissue from vital organs gathered in postmortems in thirty-three cities around the globe, from Honolulu to Cairo. Body lead appeared everywhere and was highest in industrialized areas, including the United States.

Clearly lead has been piling up in our biosphere and our bodies. The question is whether there exists a threshold below which it is harmless. Or is there a chronic, low-level plumbism which, without overt poisoning, disturbs children's behavior and learning, increases vulnerability to disease, shortens life, raises stillbirth rates, and is passed from parent to infant? Many authorities disagree, but for more than a decade opinion has shifted away from the safe-threshold idea to serious worry that low-level plumbism may create long-lasting damage.

Animal experiments show that even small amounts of TEL may impair reflexes, and several scientists fear that it affects the nervous systems and behavior of children in high-pollution areas. Dr. Herbert L. Needleman of Harvard Medical School echoes the concern of the National Academy of Sciences about airborne lead: "The high blood levels in children near smelters in El Paso and Toronto, the high tooth lead levels in children near a paint factory in Philadelphia indict airborne lead from stationary industrial sources. Is lead from a moving tailpipe somehow different?"

There is still no decisive proof that we are immediately endangered, no proof that we are not. Henry Schroeder says, "There is no National Catastrophe in the offing. There are local areas where things are serious, as there have been and will be. There is less air and water pollution per capita now than a hundred years ago, but there are more people. Our cities have been cleaning their air since 1955. . . ." But he also says that introducing TEL started "the most wide-spread pollution of the human environment that has ever occurred . . . for any toxic element." He recommends not eating vegetables grown near well-traveled roads.

Professor R. A. Kehoe sees no massive general threat from lead; his findings were among those criticized at the 1965 PHS conference. But Patterson, who studied lead in Greenland ice, argues that the American people are subjected to "chronic lead insult." He estimates that urban dwellers' body lead may now be a hundred times the natural level — in the United States, perilously close to the level defined for clinical lead poisoning. While the question is argued, we shape our health and our species' future by acting or not acting on lead pollution. And lead has had a striking history of being a more complex, serious threat to health than most people anticipated.

We need more research on the interplay of lead with calcium and other substances, inside and outside our bodies; on how bone lead can be mobilized; on lead's environmental pathways to man. We also need massive screening programs, better and cheaper tests for body lead, and education not only for the public but for health professionals. Some immediate housecleaning is also needed. A few old cities, including Boston, still have lead pipes in their water systems, supplying millions of people. Old house paint remains a threat; repainting is not protection enough, for children with pica sometimes gnaw right through all layers of paint to the wood. Improperly glazed pottery is still common. Overt poisoning still occurs too often among smelters, metal scrappers, auto repairmen, printshop workers, and residents near their plants. And of course TEL still pours into our atmosphere.

The first time a nation acted against TEL was in 1969, when Sweden's Poison Board lowered the lead limit in gasoline. Since the early 1970s, American cities, states, and federal agencies have moved to reduce or eliminate lead and other pollutants from gasoline, but no absolute national ban has resulted. At every step there has been stubborn industry resistance. In the years 1976–1980, U.S. blood lead levels decreased about one-third, as the use of TEL declined, but the additive is still in use. Complete phase-out is hopefully planned here for the 1990s, but in some parts of Europe and the rest of the world, no ban is imminent.

Argument remains over a permissible lead level. In 1973, New York City's Board of Health screened almost 125,000 children and found that 761 had alarming levels of blood lead. The next year, now conscious of silent effects from smaller amounts of lead, the city reduced its danger level by one-third. Had this standard been used in 1973, the number of seriously endangered children would have been 50 percent higher. Patterson and other scientists have long complained that permissible levels may be much too high; levels thought safe a decade or so ago now cause researchers alarm. A sharp political struggle is still going on in Washington over reducing the threshold of danger.

About a million workers remain at risk at their jobs; so do their children, who may suffer plumbism because of dust in their parents' clothing. We have said that lead can cause stillbirths and congenital malformations by affecting a man's sperm or crossing a woman's placental barrier. This became a civil rights issue in the late seventies, when it came to light that some women of childbearing age were having themselves sterilized in order to keep high-paying jobs at which they were exposed to lead.

Even with industrial exposure and TEL eliminated, lead will remain a potential hazard. Myriad demands in future technology could, as in the past, bring pervasive and pernicious environmental lead contamination. If there is a lesson in the biohistory of lead, it is how often the metal has been forgotten as a poison and then rediscovered at great cost. Lead remains in glazes, inks, toys, dust. Odd sources keep being found. Recently, acute plumbism has been traced to *azarcon,* or *greta,* a folk remedy consisting mostly of lead that is used widely in our Mexican communities and south of our border. This lethal drug can be bought in many Latin shops in American cities.

While we try to cope with the risks from lead, mercury, cadmium, arsenic, and asbestos, complex chemicals from pesticides to preservative become new causes of cancer, birth defects, and other medical misfortunes. Some half million synthetic substances have entered our biosphere since World War II, as many as one-fifth of them toxic. There are also, of course, the problems posed by radioactive wastes. Man and his inventions have always engaged in an ambivalent dance.

It is fashionable today to speak of trade-offs in environmental problems, balancing the costs and benefits of pollutants. Much technology that can poison us does bring better health, better living, and longer lives. The question is whether in this, as in advances in nuclear and biological warfare, man's presumptuous, inventive mind will overleap itself. The use and abuse of lead show that health is no simple matter of defeating once and for all a static enemy. The same lesson must be learned, as we shall see, about substances far more complex, which may change the world for our descendants.

8

The Upright, the Erotic

BIOHISTORY AND SOCIAL HISTORY

I T is one thing to call a man upright, another to say he has reverted to all fours. Upright implies morality and moderation; it suggests that in rising to our hind legs, we have abandoned doggish lusts for a posture of divine aspiration. It is a grand vision of human body and mind, this alleged ascent from rut to rectitude, but it is quite mistaken; the upright tread the path of the licentious. Upright posture has developed along with a sexual appetite and capacity unique in nature. This erotic evolution is still going on, and it may soon take incalculable turns because of widespread changes in life-styles and in contraceptive methods.

This development is very much the province of biohistory, which deals with behavior as well as health, the human species as well as its members. If there is a common human nature, it rises from a common genetic endowment. Unfortunately, this aspect of our natural history provokes as much polemical heat as does political history; it is similarly revised in waves of fashion, passion, and doctrine. Some people hate to think that they excel in "animal" urges, and that some of their intimate emotions are guided as much by the genes as by the heart. Besides, we were ill prepared to judge such matters. Our first picture of evolution came from books that compared a bat's wing, a seal's flipper, and the human hand, showing how the body adapts to different environments. The stress on comparative anatomy diverted us from seeing that behavior evolves just as the body does — that in fact the body may change *because* behavior does.

Often people aren't really arguing that the genes don't shape behavior, only that they don't shape behavior that involves their cherished convictions. Few deny that seals gotta swim and bats gotta fly; that everyone blinks at sudden noises; that some of us are born with very high or low aptitudes for balletics or mathematics. But suggest that there is some genetic basis for sex behavior, sex differences, or family formation, and debate may turn stubborn, bitter. Such thoughts threaten many people's dignity and their hopes for social justice, raising specters of racism and eugenic tyranny.

Furthermore, the very phrase genetic trait can evoke powerful feelings of giftedness or doom; desires to be like or unlike one's forebears; a longing to change or conform to society. To blame the genes seems to blame fate, and denying their power seems to assert free will. Actually, either view, taken to its logical end, is threatening. If behavior has genetic guidelines, it may resist upbringing and reasoned change, yet obey biological engineering. If upbringing and choice are stronger than the genes, the social engineering of altruists and dictators are equally possible.

Such attitudes make genetic and social determinism straw men in futile debates. Actually, modern genetics does not put full responsibility on the body physical or the body social. Clearly some traits, such as ejaculation and menstruation, are limited to one sex; others, such as aggression and nurture, occur more strongly in one sex but exist in both; still other traits, such as memory ability, seem equal in both sexes. Behavior genetics now says that in all but the most automatic physical and behavioral traits, the genes set a potential range of development, and the environment determines how far that potential is realized.

Researchers are trying to sort out the genetic and social roots of human sexuality. In judging the evidence, one must resist the tendency to load it with morality, ideology, and one's own particular experience. Psychologist Milton Diamond has given this useful caveat in matters of sex: "We must always distinguish what is from what might be or 'should' be." That is, before rejecting or embracing any picture of our sexual evolution and where it may lead, we should see clearly where we are. The first step is grasping how we became the upright and superlatively erotic creatures we are.

To begin with, one should not confuse sex and reproduction. Reproduction doesn't require sex, only the transmission of genes; the first, simplest organisms just replicated their genes and split in two. Sex arose when one cell penetrated the wall of another so that they could blend their genes and create offspring with characteristics of both. Because of spontaneous changes in each organism, no two have quite the same genetic makeup; therefore blending two sets of genes to produce a third creates greater genetic diversity than cell division. This diversity raises the potential for change in a changing environment.

Many simple organisms still reproduce asexually, but sexual reproduction became entrenched in vertebrates. So did sexual dimorphism, the existence of two forms in each species. The basic difference between the sexes remains the gametes, the egg and sperm — and the gonads that produce them — but eventually dimorphism extended to the entire reproductive system, and then to organs and behavior not directly involved in copulation. Mating had become just one moment in a long, complicated reproductive cycle with distinct roles for each partner. It might include winning a territory, establishing social rank, courtship, nesting, mating, pregnancy, giving birth, and rearing the young. Each species has its own distinctive pattern, and the variety is baroque.

Even at the simple level of coital push and pull, the diversity is florid. Despite D. H. Lawrence's assertion, the elephant is not slow to mate; he may finish copulating in ten seconds. Grizzlies take ten to sixty minutes; the South American opossum lolls in coitus for up to six hours; marsupial mice lock at the genitals for half a day. Species also vary in their number of partners and coitions. A male mouse makes several to a dozen insertions, with one or more partners, before ejaculating; a rat may reach his little nirvana only with his tenth or twelfth female. Coital positions are a study in themselves. Possums mate lying on their sides. Porcupines do, as the joke says, make love very carefully; the male stands above the female, hardly touching her except at the genitals. A female rhesus monkey must bear most of the male's weight. Humans show variety; tradition defines a gentleman as one who keeps at least half his weight on his elbows.

In lower vertebrates, sex and much other behavior are rigidly programmed by the genes, hormones, and nervous system. Frogs, for instance, reproduce through mechanisms rather like reflexes, without having to learn how. Many mammals, however, must to some degree learn to court, mate, and rear their young; anyone who has watched cats mate knows that their first attempts can be almost as clumsy as people's. Their behavior is incompletely pro-

grammed at birth; the forebrain, or cerebral cortex, has
enlarged to finish the job through learning. Humans are
nature's most radical experiment in dependence on learning, with its potential for flexibility and variety — and for
mislearning.

The shift from programming to learning was shown in
recent decades in experiments by three famous psychologists. In 1956 Alan E. Fisher injected testosterone into
different areas of rats' brains until he pinpointed the cells
in which the hormone activates aggression and sexual
arousal. That launched a new era of research, still under
way, of mapping and measuring the hormonal control of
behavior. Such research has shown that hormones from
an embryo's gonads prime its brain before birth to react
in certain typically male or female ways throughout life.

It remained to be discovered what released or activated
the hormones. During the fifties and sixties, Daniel Lehrman's detailed studies of ring doves revealed that their
reproduction depends on a chain of synchronized male
and female signals for hormone release. Each partner gives
visual or other cues that create a response in the other,
which in turn initiates the next step. For instance, a female
dove isolated in a lab will not sit on her eggs. An injection
of the hormone progesterone makes her do so, but in her
normal environment that isn't necessary. In nature she
can see her mate, and in the lab if she can do so, even
through glass that kills sounds and scents, she will incubate
her eggs. Obviously a visual cue from the male releases
progesterone in her body. Such cues pass back and forth
between mates through courtship, mating, nest building,
egg laying, incubation, and rearing the young.

In doves, these steps still proceed more or less like
reflexes; in mammals, more is required, and that became
the subject of Harry Harlow's famous experiments with

rhesus monkeys in the fifties and sixties. He began by raising infant monkeys in isolation with surrogate mothers — wire dummies with wooden heads and feeding bottles. At first, Harlow was trying to learn what binds rhesus infant and mother; the initial results led to many ingenious experiments about primate sociosexual development. Infant monkeys deprived of real mothers behaved much like autistic human children, withdrawn and self-destructive. Their social and sexual growth was stunted, so as adults they sometimes showed sexual arousal but didn't know how to act with other monkeys. The males would grab a female and thrust futilely at her back or side. The females wouldn't present their hindquarters or accept a male's weight. Harlow said, "Their hearts were in the right place, but nothing else was . . . we had developed not a breeding colony but a brooding colony."

With great effort and patience, Harlow got a few of the unmothered females to become mothers themselves. Not one of their infants would have survived without his intervention. The mothers, unable to give what they had never experienced, relentlessly ignored or attacked them. However, some of the mothers had second pregnancies, and the results were better. Even as adults, they learned through experience to make up for their early deficits in development. This is a beautiful example of evolution's gamble on the risks of learning rather than the inflexible certainty of programming: it allows for change and improvement on the past.

Whatever the gap between doves and monkeys, there is a still greater gulf between them and ourselves, with our vast dependence on learning. Partly because of learning, partly because of our particular sexual circuitry, we are by far the sexiest of species. After all, sex takes up little of most creatures' time; the seasons bring a brief annual burst of sex, perhaps lasting only days. Even in species that mate in any season, only after a female has borne and raised a litter does she again become estrous, or sexually receptive, and send arousing signals to males. Some captive and domesticated animals do seem to act like repeat sex offenders, but a careful observer usually finds only fragments of mating behavior, such as mounting without coitus to express dominance, touching the genitals without proceeding to orgasm, or presenting the hindquarters in response to a friendly touch.

No mammal matches our incessant eroticism. None, except perhaps dolphins, are so sexually active and excitable all through the year. Certainly none other mates during menstruation, pregnancy, and lactation, before fertility begins and after it fades. None choose oral-genital or anal-genital intercourse; none regularly masturbate to orgasm; none, despite myths to the contrary, show exclusive homosexuality as adults. By comparison, rabbits and baboons are abstemious.

Humans have also developed unique sex organs and unique ways of using them. The vaginal opening has shifted from the back toward the front of the body, making us the only land mammals that can and usually do mate face to face. Most female mammals, though active in courtship, merely accept a male's thrusting; women not only abet coitus, they actively aid it. Perhaps distinctive as well are the wide frequency of female orgasm and direct use of the clitoris to attain it. The clitoris is the only organ, in either sex, that exists solely to provide sexual pleasure. Although the clitoris exists in many mammals, coitus from behind probably gives it even less stimulation than coitus face to face. And I know only one reliable account of a female primate, living under abnormal zoo conditions, touching her clitoris to the point of orgasm. Female orgasm does seem to happen in some species, such as cats and rabbits, but the usual signs of peak body tension followed by relaxation are rare even in higher primates. The clitoris is doubtless more than decorative in animals that have it, but it may usually give pleasure without orgasm, as is often true in humans.

Our sexual uniqueness goes beyond the genitals. Women are the only female mammals with round, protruding breasts and, as far as we know, with erotically sensitive nipples. We are uniquely hairless among primates; some guess that this was an adaptation of African prehumans to help regulate body temperature. Whatever its origin, hairlessness has allowed the entire skin to become a secondary sex organ; it is both erotically sensitive and an erotic visual and tactile stimulus. Hairlessness may also be a sign of neoteny, the persistence of childish traits into adulthood. Neoteny is more pronouned in humans than any other species, as it aids the process of developing through learning rather than programming. Such neotenic traits as the persistence in adults of curiosity and playfulness may also have helped create our vast elaboration of sex into a nonstop, nonreproductive game.

Certainly no other species shows such sexual variety among individuals and groups. Some people have coitus once or twice a day, some almost never. Some take only minutes at mating, others spend hours at foreplay alone. There are societies where polygamy is forbidden, others where it is idealized; some where women do not reveal their faces, others where they wear only tiny pubic aprons; some where almost no one has had homosexual experience, others where most men have had at least a little; some where girls' labia are sewn together to ensure virginity at marriage, others where they begin premarital coitus at ten.

Finally, no other creature has such long-lasting, extensive, and complex sexual and family bonds. Even many
primates' mateships last only a season, days, or hours; sex
ends when the female becomes pregnant, and usually the
mates' bond ends when sex ends. Human society is based
on the family, the addition of the father to the ancient
bond of mother and child, and the addition of other kin
such as grandparents, uncles, and aunts. Not all societies
share the West's ideal of exclusive, lifelong monogamy,
but all recognize and support a lasting tie between biological parents, their offspring, and a wider family network.

We do not know just when and how humans became
the sexiest species. Archaeologists, anthropologists, and
students of human and animal behavior are beginning to
trace the path and relate it to other changes in body, mind,
and behavior. Many now agree that the starting point was
our simian ancestors' gradual descent from the trees to
the grassy savannas of Africa, perhaps starting as long as
twenty million years ago. They eventually became the only
primates to stand fully erect and walk entirely on their
hind limbs. With their hands free, their thumbs enlarged
for better tool using. As the forebrain grew, and of ne-
cessity the skull, the female pelvis widened to give the
infant's head safe passage during birth. The mouth and
throat altered to allow an enormous variety of sounds.
Prehumans became more dependent on animal food than
most primates, and this changed their dentition and their
behavior.

By two or three million years ago, our ancestors were
using rudimentary tools and perhaps starting to live as
modern hunter-gatherers do. They or later prehumans
probably formed male groups for hunting and defense,
while women worked at gathering and other tasks that

could safely be done with infants and toddlers in tow. Sexual dimorphism and the sexual division of labor probably increased. The emerging human species, though predatory and aggressive, was deeply social and nurturing; they had to be, for the larger forebrain and extended helplessness of the young required years of physical and emotional care. Now, perhaps, came a florid growth of eroticism, as a sort of glue binding couples through long habits of pleasure, and as a vehicle for such nonsexual needs as touch and reassurance. Since sex carries a potential for competition and conflict, the growth of eroticism also required social controls on sex. Perhaps awareness of the controls has made people assume that those controls, rather than sex, were the hallmark of humanity.

We may never know in just what order prehumans became fully upright and developed tool-using, speech, intelligence, foresight, and a wild flowering of sex and relationships. Probably they grew in tandem, reinforcing each other. Together they led to greater face-to-face communication in sex, an evolutionary shift perhaps still under way. There have been similar, instructive changes in two other primates, the gelada baboon and mandrill baboon, which communicate sexually face-to-face for quite different reasons.

Baboons, one of the few ground-dwelling primates, mate with the male entering from behind. The female gelada signals that she is estrous by developing great rosy patches on her rump and vivid marks about the vulva. Because baboons spend so much time squatting rather than on all fours, these signals are often invisible. Evolution has ingeniously provided; the vulvar design waxes and wanes in duplicate on her chest along with the sexual cycle. A similar frontward shift of sexual signals occurs in the male mandrill. He has a red penis and blue scrotal patches; like the female gelada's genital signals, these are hidden when he squats. To make his sexual message always clear, he duplicates it on his face, with a bright-red nose and blue cheeks.

Many creatures, from tropical fish to baboons, send sexual signals only at mating time. Since we are potentially erotic all the time, our signals appear permanently at puberty. In us, as in most mammals, the initial signals come from females, and males respond more than they to visual erotic cues. Therefore the most striking signals exist chiefly or solely in women, and many are frontal duplications of ones that used to come from the rear.

We are the only primates with high, rounded buttocks; we are also the only ones with round, prominent breasts. The roundness of the breasts has no known function except to mimic the ancient primate signal of the hindquarters. The attractiveness of rosy cheeks, breasts, and buttocks may all echo our ancestors' arousing red rumps. This theory is supported by our unique erotizing of the breasts; in keeping with our species' luxuriant sexuality, men have rudimentary nipples that may be erotically sensitive. We are also the only primates with thick red lips, and these, like the breasts, have been erotized; they may echo the pink, fleshy vulva. It has been guessed that underarm hair mimics the arousing pubic thatch. Our full red lips, bare skin, and axillary hair may not have developed solely as sexual signals, but they have certainly come to act as such.

Such shifts are new in evolutionary terms, but another part of our sexuality still follows a very old scenario. Ethologists call it courtship; most other people call it flirting and seduction. The steps of this mating dance are basically the same in most higher species, and as Lehrman showed, they proceed through genetically and hormonally controlled actions and reactions. A perfect example, with great relevance for humans, is the courting of black-headed gulls, described in fine detail by Nobel laureate Niko Tinbergen.

In gulls, as in many higher species, males as a group are bigger, stronger, and more aggressive than females. At breeding season, a male's aggression runs especially high, for he will have to protect his territory, mate, and offspring from rivals and predators. Having established a territory, he defends it against all comers; but now, having proven his fitness as a mate, he is still more ready for war than for love. The female will have to remotivate the bellicose male; accept the vulnerability of coitus (to most creatures, being touched means danger, attack); draw on her nurturing qualities to raise the young.

To these gulls, both a direct stare and the sight of their species' dark face mask are challenges; therefore when a female enters a male's territory, she does so with head averted. Now both will court through ritualized behavior, acts used outside their original contexts with a formalized quality that makes the new meanings clear. The male struts and puffs himself up, things he does in times of danger to look bigger and more threatening; by averting his face and modifying the gestures, he signals that he isn't really ready to fight, merely displaying his better self. The female responds with ritualized gestures of appeasement and flight.

To become more intimate, the pair proceed from their initial mock aggression and appeasement to gestures of nurture. Some species do so through grooming, cleaning each other's fur or feathers. Gulls use ritualized food-begging and feeding. A gull chick stimulates its parents to feed it with a specific food-begging noise; courting adults use it as well, but the context and an added head-tossing motion show that the message is not literally "Feed me" but "Care for me as you would a helpless chick." This evokes both gulls' nurture, reduces the difference in dominance, and draws them closer. The male may actually feed the female; if he does, they are almost sure to mate.

Often people smile when watching such animal courtship, for it seems to parody the course of human courting from strutting and coyness to intimacy. Of course it is not parody but the evolutionary paradigm of our own behavior. The major difference between us and other creatures is the addition of language, our unique and most extensive communication system, which becomes a vehicle for assertion, appeasement, nurture, and intimacy. A courting couple talk more to create closeness than to exchange information, and ethologist Desmond Morris has aptly called their chatter "grooming talk."

The basic language of courtship remains nonverbal, and in any public place you can see people repeat the gulls' mating dance. It usually seems to begin with a man communicating authority or dominance by his posture, standing or sitting straight, perhaps with his arms folded or chest thrown out. He draws close to the woman, gives a challenging look, or starts talking to her. Actually, he rarely does so unless she has already taken the first step — the equivalent of entering his territory. She may draw near or take a position that allows his approach, engage him with a smile or word, or act as if he had already made an overture. Her physical message is unmistakable; she holds her body straight and her head high, brushes back her hair or straightens some item of clothing, perhaps arches her back to display buttocks and breast. She returns his glance and then averts her head or lowers her eyes; she may smile at his words and then cover her mouth with her hands.

Such behavior is not learned but innate, and often unconscious; people would be shocked to see it in films of their own actions. Even little girls who were born blind often respond to compliments by smiling and then averting their heads and covering their faces with their hands. Eventually courtship escalates to touching, first briefly and lightly, then longer and more intimately. There may even be courting with gifts of food; when a man offers drinks or dinner or a woman volunteers to cook, the gesture is usually more than culinary. If a gull had a forebrain, it would want to smile in recognition.

We are only starting to create a human ethology, the observation of human behavior outside laboratories and testing rooms. Already that study is revealing more about erotic interactions. Some fascinating research is now being completed by Timothy Perper, an expert in genetics and animal sex behavior who turned to studying human sexuality. Over several years he watched hundreds upon hundreds of people engaged in flirting and pick-ups in bars, from small-town and neighborhood hangouts to big-city singles bars. Regardless of the setting or the words, men and women went through the same courtship dance, in ways that defy some people's expectations.

Tradition claims that men start the courtship dance, primarily through words, and press it on decreasingly reluctant women. Perper found that in humans, as in gulls and baboons, females start, guide, and direct courtship, least of all through words. Almost invariably, he observed, a couple talk only after the woman has drawn close or somehow invited the man's approach. He also found that as flirtation proceeds, a couple sitting side by side turn slowly, over a period of up to an hour, until they fully face each other. Then they begin touching; again, it is usually the woman who acts first, placing her palm on the man's forearm or chest or brushing against his body while seeming to turn to look elsewhere. Only then does the man touch in return. Then gradually the couple's body movements synchronize. They lift their glasses simultaneously, shift weight together, sway to the music together. They are quite literally in a courtship dance.

Perper saw that any step along the way may seem casual, even accidental, when it happens, but the same sequence occurs in virtually every successful encounter. Just as in gulls, it proceeds only if each stage is completed properly; each partner must accept and reciprocate the other's gesture or the dance shuffles to a halt. Perper's research was in bars, and that may mislead some people about its probable universality. Not all bar pickups are for instant sex, and even in more "respectable" settings, the courtship process seems basically the same.

This research is a humbling lesson to advocates of total honesty who deplore flirting's "artificiality" and "manipulation." They prefer that we relentlessly reveal our blemished selves to our blemished neighbors. But we reveal ourselves eventually, and hurrying the moment may not turn strangers into friends. Courtship's chatter, grooming, and preening are, to truly rational minds, inane, but they rise from our deepest instincts. They aim not at honing minds but at finding fit, safe partners for mating (to all creatures, mating is a moment of complete physical vulnerability). Information and revelation are more safely traded after intimacy has grown; for that, the ancient signals of the smile, touch, and pointless remark serve best. Anyway, even champions of pitiless sincerity end up courting like gulls, unaware.

Most of those urging honesty are probably men. When Perper interviewed people he had observed, he found the men stunningly unaware of courtship's steps and of who had taken them in which order; they called the whole thing "magic" or "chemistry." Virtually every woman had been conscious of each step and the strategy behind it. They knew that although courtship demands men's shows of assertion, it depends more on women's choices and initiatives. To male scientists, this was an old but often ignored discovery; Darwin wrote in 1874 that sexual selection results from females' reproductive choices. People who don't see bar pickups as reproductive choices ignore that the same courtship programming is probably triggered in most erotic or even potentially erotic encounters, and forget the extent to which bars have replaced such traditional places for meeting mates as churches and clubs. After all, most spouses were once flirting partners; most were pickups, though they may not use that term; and today the majority were once lovers.

None of this surprises women; they and a few wise men have always known that in mating, women are the choosers and movers, while men can only enter doors left ajar for them. Both sexes, however, may wonder why, if courtship's steps are innate, it often fails. In higher species, most of all in ours, one must learn to perform the steps deftly and in sequence. Flirting and seduction are the last sociosexual skills many people master, and some hardly learn them at all. Courtship demands normal animal sensitivity and normal animal courage; almost any fear, fantasy, or inhibition can get in the way.

Sometimes failures rise from social differences. In some American subcultures, men strut like peacocks and show open, lavish erotic interest; the women preen and display like jungle birds. In other groups, the gestures, though basically the same, are understated. When people from different backgrounds meet, one may give a word or touch the other thinks too directly sexual too early; that threatens the necessary sense of intimacy and security. Or the dance may falter and fail because one partner sends signals the other finds tentative, responses that seem ambiguous.

More often, courtship failures have psychological roots. Some people, lacking self-esteem, expect rejection and retreat from courting. Others are convinced, realistically or not, that they are unattractive, and through self-contempt assume that there is something wrong with anyone who would settle for them. Others freeze, afraid their loneliness and need will show and make them seem ridiculous. Still others fear that their sexual fantasies can be divined, and that the fantasies are repulsive. Some see all relationships as power struggles and fear becoming a master or slave. Those who feel that any assertion and sexuality are vaguely wrong or dangerous may vacillate between social talk and mating talk, and send a confusion of sexual and nonsexual signals with their bodies. The other person, not knowing which message to believe most, becomes wary and backs away.

Whatever their sources, the barriers to human courtship are often essentially those which keep gulls asunder. Like so many creatures, gulls won't mate unless the male acts more assertive, the female less challenging. Despite complex psychological and social variations, people usually follow the same pattern. Men tend to be turned off by women they see as challenging, women by men who seem indecisive. Courting signals are sometimes subtle, even paradoxical; a man's aloofness may be a gesture of power, a woman's challenge her invitation to be psychically outwrestled. Still, the basic evolutionary pattern holds, and couples who to some degree violate it often do so at some emotional or sexual cost.

Gulls must master these problems only briefly, once a year. Our long bonds and strong eroticism make the pleasures and problems of courting and mating a permanent part of life. A couple who live and make love together experience daily the interplay of dominance, intimacy, nurture, courtship, and mating, and the neurohormonal signals they involve. This makes human life complicated enough; we are complicating it further, perhaps altering our future, with chemical contraceptives, prescribed drugs, and mood-altering substances. The effects of oral contraceptives are especially important, and they remain relatively ignored by society and science.

Chemical contraceptives are possible because of the peculiar human cycles of sex and reproduction. Men's fertility and sex behavior have no cycle; women's sexuality has two. Menstruation, which exists only in primates, is a change in the uterus; ovulation, a process of the ovaries, occurs roughly between menses. These cycles, synchronized by neurohormonal feedbacks, involve shifting balances of many hormones, especially estrogen and progesterone. Estrogen, which primes a woman's sexuality, peaks during ovulation; progesterone, which tends to muffle sexuality, peaks near menses. In nonhuman primates, females become estrous, arouse males, and mate only when fertile, at ovulation. We have weakened but not broken the old link between sex and fertility.

Women may become pregnant at any time, even during menses, but are most fertile at ovulation, and that is when they have sex most often. As a group, they desire sex more during ovulation, engage more often then in coitus and masturbation, and are most often orgasmic. They are least turned on sexually, and least active, during menses. There are individual exceptions; obviously women do not leap into bed when ovulating or flee it when menstruating. (Also, because of complex hormonal shifts, some women have secondary peaks of arousal just before or after menses.) Many women say sex depends on the right man and the right mood, but studies of large populations show that the right man and right mood appear most often during ovulation.

These hormonal cycles have other effects with sexual consequences. Women feel pain least at ovulation, most during menstruation. They smell, see, hear, and taste with greater sensitivity around ovulation, less acutely during menses. At ovulation they tend to feel more satisfied with themselves, more effervescent, better able to cope with life. Menses may bring anxiety, fatigue, depression, irritability, low self-esteem, and physical symptoms from abdominal cramps to water retention. Such problems afflict one-third to two-thirds of American women.

Some women are barely affected by their menses and doubt those who complain of severe tension, depression, and pain. Some people have downplayed the problems for fear that it will be used to justify traditional job barriers. However unfair certain job barriers, it is equally unfair to deny millions of women's discomfort. A half-century of extensive research has clearly linked the so-called premenstrual tension syndrome with statistical increases in women's accidents, physical and mental ills, and poor performance in examinations and athletics. Some recent studies implicate prostaglandins, hormonelike substances produced in the brain and other parts of the body. In any case, the sexual implications are clear. A comfortable, confident woman is more likely to want to mate, and to find a mate, than one who is temporarily depressed, tense, and in pain.

Another time when estrogen decreases and progesterone rises is pregnancy. As pregnancy advances, sexual interest and activity wane, orgasmic response dwindles. A survey of sixty preliterate societies showed that coitus became less frequent during pregnancy in all the cultures, and it virtually ended in three-quarters of them. In those societies, as in ours, many people say they avoid sex for fear of harming the fetus, but today the medical consensus is that such risks are low (except perhaps for a matter of weeks before delivery). The attitude may actually rationalize a physical change. As pregnancy proceeds and progesterone rises, women, not surprisingly, become preoccupied, fatigued, and less interested in sex. One needn't be an ethologist to presume that a tired, turned-off woman turns off her mate.

Knowledge of how one person's hormones influence others is still dismally thin, but there are strong hints. Women friends who live together have been observed to synchronize their menstrual periods. A study of couples shows that men's testosterone, which causes sexual arousal, peaks soon after their partners have ovulated, at the height of their fertility. Like other mammals, we may send and receive myriad visual, olfactory, and behavioral cues at highs and lows of fertility. The matter is complicated by the fact that behavior influences hormones. The tension of anticipating an examination can delay a woman's ovulation or menstruation and raise a man's testosterone level. We have only recently developed laboratory techniques that allow us to map the interplay of hormones and behavior, and much research lies ahead.

Without benefit of such research, we have begun to change millions of people's bodies, minds, and behavior with chemical contraceptives. These were developed after World War II through ingenious research and experiment. The only known substances that reduced men's fertility were antitestosterone agents; these also caused impotence and feminization, so they prevented pregnancy only by preventing sex. Research therefore had to focus on blocking ovulation, menstruation, or implantation. The best solution seemed to be a pill containing estrogen and progesterone, which gave a woman's body a false message that she was pregnant. A woman who is pregnant stops ovulating, so that her body will not accept further impregnations, and she stops menstruating as well.

In the early years of testing and using the pill, it became clear that many women suffered such signs of pregnancy as nausea, dizziness, headaches, depression, swollen and tender breasts, weight gain, flattened emotions, and decreased sexual interest and response. Researchers juggled the dosages and the balance of hormones, and the pill improved. Soon it was being casually prescribed for acne and painful periods; some women even took it merely to avoid the inconvenience of menses.

In 1968, in a little-noticed scientific paper, Masters and Johnson mentioned that some women using the pill felt reduced sexual interest and difficulty reaching orgasm. A few subsequent researchers agreed; a few others found sex unchanged or slightly increased in pill users. The issue drew little public attention. At the time, I was beginning a series of sex-research projects that required taking hundreds of exhaustive sexual biographies. I kept hearing stories from women and their partners that convinced me there was a quiet epidemic of sexual, emotional, and marital problems caused by the pill.

Many women told only of dwindling sexual interest and loss of orgasm; some described severe physical and emotional changes as well. Since the problems had appeared gradually, few women linked them to the pill until ceasing to take it brought dramatic relief. For instance, one woman said: "After a year or so on the pill, I felt irritable and distant all the time; it was as if I was always slightly under water. My husband and I were quarreling a lot, first because I was depressed, then about sex. I started to have pounding headaches as I became sexually excited, and the more excited I became, the worse the pain got. Finally I would scream from pain instead of reaching orgasm." The symptoms so frightened her that she went through months of tests with internists and neurologists. At a loss, still testing, the doctors told her to stop all medication. She was taking none but the pill, and when she put it aside, her complaints vanished. She found it interesting, but her doctors, she said, were not intrigued.

After hearing many such stories, I began discussing them with other sex researchers. Some gave confirmation. An eminent psychiatrist said he had seen the pill's effects many times: "In fact, I've just finished treating a couple, two young doctors, whose problem came from the pill. She stopped responding sexually and became depressed and agitated. They assumed it was psychological and saw a marriage counselor, but that didn't help. They were on the verge of separating, and the counselor referred them to me. As I followed various leads, I suggested that she stop taking the pill. She did, and their problems virtually went away."

Research on this subject required controlled medical experiments, so I sought doctors interested in doing them with me or on their own. Some were interested in the matter of the pill, sex, and relationships when I mentioned it, but no one was interested enough. There has always been a gap between researchers interested in the body and those interested in emotions. Women kept telling me how their doctors avoided this subject. Almost no one I interviewed had been warned of possible sexual and emotional effects; no one had been asked about them in follow-up exams. Those who complained were told the problems would pass, were unrelated to the pill, or should be taken to a psychotherapist. Doctors in sexology were more interested than those in other fields, but less than one would have expected. I became convinced that if so many people were bent on avoiding a subject, it must be especially important.

Oddly, some of the avoidance may have risen from bad press the pill was receiving on other counts. Then, in the early seventies, the popular wisdom from corner bars to medical seminars held that the pill had made adolescent mating grunts the Western world's major background noise. While an editor at *Newsweek,* I suggested and wrote an article disproving that myth. Kinsey had already shown that fear of pregnancy didn't prevent sex, just made people worry about it; furthermore, cheap contraceptives had been available for a century. Now research from several clinics confirmed what common sense should have foretold. Almost no girls decided to begin coitus because of the pill; they started sex, worried about pregnancy, and then sought the pill. Some couples had sex a bit more often because of the pill, but they had been at it already.

I was fascinated to see other editors' disbelief, then their grudging assent when they saw the evidence, then their reluctance to pursue the subject. A cynic might suspect that it was hotter journalism to say the pill turned people on than that it did nothing or turned them off. Yet I think those editors, like many of their readers, were reacting with a genuine and visceral will to disbelieve. A whole decade, while sometimes deploring an alleged sexual revolution, didn't want its fantasies contradicted by facts or complexities.

Meanwhile, many public critics of the pill had appeared, some virtually making careers on possible links between the pill and embolism, cancer, hypertension, vaginal disorders. Some of the fears were quite justified, others little or not at all. Few of these writers, busy with their particular crusades, wanted to ponder problems less lethal but far more common. A few did show concern over studies in England and Scandinavia which showed that up to one-third of women on the pill suffered some degree of depression. Still, the effects of the pill on sex and relationships were no one's chief concern. I had stumbled on a compelling subject that violated popular fantasies, paled beside related disasters, and suggested such unwelcome headlines as PILL SLOWS SEXUAL REVOLUTION. Regardless of doctors and the press, women kept telling me that the pill seriously affected their sexuality, emotions, and marriages.

In 1973, as editor of another magazine, I asked several people to take on the subject in depth; it was difficult to find someone interested and competent. Finally it was done by Lionel Tiger, an eminent sociologist well schooled in ethology and the physical roots of behavior. His essay probed the subject as deeply as I had hoped. In fact, it crystallized thoughts I had merely been groping for, and it shifted my attention to the long-term evolutionary effects of the pill.

The pill, said Tiger, was probably the most powerful, influential drug ever given to so many people, "possibly more coercive than the strongest puritanism." He pointed out that researchers Richard Michael and Doris Zumpe in London had given the pill to rhesus monkeys and found that males were less eager to mate with them than with other females; when the males did, they took longer to reach orgasm. There was no research on how men reacted to women on the pill, but it's a logical guess that they might be less turned on by their mates, more turned on by other women, and that their mates might react to this in turn.

Hormones and behavior, Tiger pointed out, play a role not only between the sexes but between women and other women, children, and workmates. Again, it remained to be learned just how, but it was ironic that just as so many women were reaching for new freedom and opportunity, perhaps using the pill as a way to do so, some ended up shackled by depression, zestlessness, and low self-esteem.

Tiger did not dwell in detail on the pill's possible effects on women in courting situations, seeking mates. Does a physiologically pregnant woman make different choices? Do the men she meets? Considering the many subtleties of personality and behavior involved in every pairing, there must be differences when one partner is in an altered state of body and mind. Therefore Tiger was doubtless right in saying the pill might be a silent bomb ticking away for women and all those around them. When we experiment with emotion and sexuality, we experiment with our species' future. Furthermore, we have a stake in the relatively new and fragile development of a deep, long bond between men and their mates and children. Considering this stake in harmony between the sexes and generations, we seem to be playing with it lightly.

In the decade since that essay appeared, sexologists have given more attention to such rare deviations as transsexualism than to the effects of chemical contraceptives on the emotions of millions of women around the world, and on their mates, children, and friends. Today when I discuss the matter with researchers and clinicians, many say that improvements in oral contraceptives now minimize side effects. Women continue to tell me that depression, headaches, sexual dysfunction, and marital battles end when they give up the pill. Some speak of the effect of feeling "self-sterilized." Meanwhile, researchers who have not fully comprehended the effects of the pill on women prepare to market a pill for men. They have been developing agents that block male fertility without killing libido or causing feminization, or so preliminary reports have said. But considering the extraordinary insensitivity to the pill's effects on women, the avoidance of the problems it has caused, one must wonder whether researchers are watching closely enough for similar effects of any chemical contraceptive on men.

If chemical contraceptives alone were affecting people's sexual, emotional, and marital lives, one could embark on a simple crusade. However, medical and pharmaceutical progress have unleashed an increasing number of drugs with similar influences. Any drug that affects blood pressure or the nervous system should be suspected of potentially influencing moods and sexuality. Some common drugs for reducing hypertension produce depression and impotence in many men, and no one knows how many suffer milder but significant effects. Sexual problems have been ascribed to medications for ills from cardiac arrhythmia to worm infestations. Psychotropic drugs such as tranquilizers, relaxants, antidepressants, and antipsychotic drugs enhance some people's sexuality but decrease libido, potence, and orgasm in others. At least as many people's moods, sexuality, and relationships are probably influenced by these drugs as by chemical contraceptives.

Many people take illicit psychotropic drugs, such as heroin and amphetamine, that in high doses eventually depress sexuality and have strong effects on emotions and behavior. Marijuana is milder and far more widely used; its effects are still poorly understood. Some people find that marijuana enhances their sexual pleasure or deinhibits them; others find that it reduces sexual interest and response. One study about a decade ago showed that prolonged marijuana use by men decreased their production of sperm and testosterone, though apparently without changing their sex behavior. Other studies showed decreased sexual activity with prolonged use of marijuana; still others showed increased probability of female orgasm. These experiments were just the first bits of a much-needed mosaic of evidence; then in 1977 Congress denied the granting of funds to study marijuana's effects on sex. Congress didn't stop sex or the use of marijuana, but it has kept their mutual effects mere guesswork. Marijuana remains one of the most widely used drugs in our society, and it promises to continue to be.

Marijuana, psychotropic drugs, all mood-altering substances, raise the same question as the chemical contraceptive pill. If people go about their lives with altered moods and altered sexuality, do they attract and choose different mates and live out their mateships and other relationships differently? Knowing what we do about courtship and the hormonal basis of behavior, we must presume the answer is yes. We are therefore watching biohistory in the making, on a grave and grand scale. Perhaps historians, physicians, and behavioral scientists will finally get interested after they can actually see dramatic aftereffects.

We said that in becoming upright, humans developed the potential to be perpetually erotic, yet in their sexual variety have maintained many basic courting and mating patterns of their evolutionary ancestors. In those distant ancestors, male orgasm evolved to reinforce the pleasure of coitus and ejaculation; female orgasm was not necessary, but seems a more recent — and therefore more fragile — development that can be cultivated or depressed by social and psychological influences. In both sexes, the great expansion of eroticism creates a pleasure bond that helps hold couples together through the longest child-rearing period in nature. This promotes a long involvement of men with their mates and offspring, also a relatively new event in mammalian life.

All of these developments suggest a picture of a species still in the process of complex and sweeping evolutionary change. Many of the hottest debates today about sex, relationships, marriage, and child-rearing involve this change; our species may still be in some problematical transition stage, groping toward better adaptations. In the midst of all this, we are chemically altering the process in ways we cannot even guess at. One of the most intriguing questions is why so few people are interested.

EPILOGUE

The Limping Ape

BIOHISTORY'S FUTURE

REGRESSIVE evolution is an arguable theory, but it tickles my imagination. I hope that if it turns out to be wrong, something equally quirky and satisfying will take its place. The idea is sufficiently paradoxical to seem true to life, and it fits much of our recent knowledge of history, health, disease, and adaptation. I suspect it hasn't found more support in the United States because at first glance it lacks that optimistic sense of progress we prefer in our past and future.

This optimism is in tune with the legacy of Darwin's age, which fervently thought nature had decreed orderly progress in science, society, and all life forms. Evolution seemed a series of forward steps, each species supplanting its predecessors by ingenious improvements and greater complexity. It was not only the fittest that survived in species from ferns to gorillas but the better, the brighter. Humans, of course, were the best, the brightest, the most ingeniously complex of all. Intense argument continued about just how evolutionary change took place, from broad ecological balance to details of genetic mechanisms. With the breaking of the genetic code in recent decades, the mechanisms are better known, but each discovery has raised new questions, and the controveries are more complicated and intense than ever. The expanding fossil record of early humans and humanlike species has brought the same growth in information and dispute.

One of the more intriguing byways in all this theory is the concept of regressive evolution, laid out in 1970 by psychiatrist David Jonas and anthropologist Doris Klein. Dr. Jonas had worked in neurology and tropical medicine before becoming a psychiatrist, and he was intensely interested in the animal roots of human behavior. Doris Klein had been trained in cultural and physical anthropology. In their book *Man-Child,* they said that nature only seems to progress in an unbroken triumph of successful, more complex forms. One reason this had often been overlooked was the traditional attitude toward the subject, which tended to deny backward or sideward evolutionary changes. Another was that most evolutionary failures, from disastrous mutations to subspecies with one fatal flaw, weren't around long enough to leave a fossil record. Even among the successful, long-lasting forms of life, said Jonas and Klein, evolution was not always a straight march from fitter to fittest, and humans are the best possible example. This is not to say that human evolution was degenerative, but that it began with disaster and proceeded by ingenious use of the wreckage. The crucial trait was neoteny, the persistence of childlike traits into adulthood.

More than a half-century ago, Dutch anatomist Ludwig Bolk pointed out striking resemblances between the adult human and the chimpanzee just before birth — hairlessness, roundheadedness, small teeth, flatness of face, absence of bony brow ridges, thin nails, and dozens of other details. These traits all fade in the chimp as it matures, but they remain to some degree in humans throughout life. "Physically," said Bolk, "man is thus a sexually mature primate fetus." Jonas and Klein say that this isn't because apes descended from a more human-looking ancestor, but because humans keep their primate fetal and infant qualities.

In behavior as well, humans resemble newborn apes more than they resemble adult apes. In chapter 8, we said how extreme human neoteny is, and how basic to human nature. It exists to some extent in many primates and sea mammals, such as chimps and dolphins, but in no creature nearly as much as in man. At all ages, humans keep much of the playful, exploratory, inventive capacity that kittens, pups, and even young primates pretty much outgrow. These qualities allow humans, a species without powerful offensive or defensive physical equipment, their best chance to adapt and survive.

Neoteny, then, is an apparent backward step in body and behavior that enabled our forebears to learn, change, and dominate their environment. Jonas and Klein say that neoteny tends to come to the fore when a species faces a survival crisis, and every ounce of adaptive capacity must be called on. They speculate that the crisis which made humans so extraordinarily neotenous was the one they think brought our ancestors down from the trees and pushed them upright — a violent pandemic of some blood-borne viral disease that almost wiped them out.

Viruses are the subject of as much research and changing theory as evolution. One must specialize in the field and read heaps of journals each week to keep from making statements that are mistaken or, at best, out of date. I think it is safe, though, to call a virus a large, complex molecule resembling the chains of protein and nucleic acid in a cell's chromosomes. A virus invades a cell, enters its nucleus, feeds, and reproduces; in the process, it may cause mutations or genetic recombinations in the host that can be passed on to future generations. This has led some scientists to speak of viruses as being, in effect, free-floating genes. Furthermore, viruses themselves can undergo mutations, making possible a vast variety of subtle genetic interactions with their hosts.

Viruses thrive especially well in parts of the body that are richly supplied with blood, such as the midbrain. The viruses causing measles, rabies, herpes simplex, polio, and encephalitis can and often do inflame the brain. The short-term effects may be weakness, apathy, and irritability. Long term, there may be paralysis or brain damage; until recently, viral brain infections left many people disabled, severely crippled, or with emotional and intellectual deficits. Such common childhood viral diseases as rubella and encephalitis are probably still responsible for a great deal of mental retardation and emotional disturbance.

Given this information, imagine a viral pandemic, a cycle of recurring infections like polio or encephalitis, striking monkeys or apes adapted to living in trees. If the disease was new to the species, the death rate and crippling would be enormous. The few survivors, their motor abilities savaged by disease, could no longer swing about in the trees. Weakened, they would have to descend to the ground and try desperately to survive there. Such epidemics may have occurred many times during primate history; only once, say Jonas and Klein, would a handful of handicapped survivors have had to succeed to start the trend of evolution toward human beings.

Perhaps at first only a few of these primates managed to get by precariously, barely managing to feed themselves, escape predators, and reproduce. Their descendants would make a marginal adaptation, future generations a more successful one, with rapid changes in behavior, anatomy, and immunity patterns — helped, perhaps, by a few lucky virus-induced mutations. Trying to adapt to a new ecological niche, they would capitalize on the flexible ways of youth to compensate for their physical weakness, drawing on their inventive, exploratory behavior to the utmost. If the results helped them survive, the neotenous traits would become part of the gene pool of the emerging new species. "It may be a distressing thought," say Jonas and Klein, "but these sickly primates were surely the forerunners of man."

Social scientist Lionel Tiger has objected that this sounds like a primate version of *Lord of the Flies,* with virus-crippled primates staggering their way to becoming a new species, thanks to a wealth of lucky mutations and a regression to more infantile traits. There are no end of objections and alternative theories. However, Jonas and Klein back up their thesis with strong, detailed arguments about the nervous and hormonal system and about viral infections. They profess that they are playfully juggling a wide range of evidence and offer only a theory, a proposition to be proven true or not true. But it is especially interesting for its use of ideas too often lacking in evolutionary theories.

Their theory does not assume consistent moves from strength to strength, which is as much a moral conviction as a scientific principle. The regressive theory allows for sideward or backward evolutionary trends (which we saw in the shift of one treponemal infection to another, both "up" and "down" the evolutionary ladder). It suggests why our progenitors came down from the trees to the ground; the conventional theories are not, to my knowledge, backed by any more evidence than the regressive theory is. It helps explain why neoteny became so big and distinctive a part of human development. It draws on something we see often in life, less often in theory — creatures building on disabilities to readapt. It gives bio-cataclysm a proper place in the tens of millions of years of primate evolution; epidemics and pandemics must have occurred many times, with enormous effects. It even suggests answers to other questions evolutionists have puzzled over, such as the sudden disappearance of the Neander-thalers; the answer may simply have been a pandemic zoonosis. The traditional explanations for too much of human development have been a sort of ecological fine tuning — without epidemics, without the unexpected, without the normal portion of disaster, surprise, and paradox we observe in life today.

The regressive theory also suggests something about the biofuture. Today we cure or prevent childhood viral diseases from rubella to polio (without, at least as far as we know, continually creating minor genetic effects through vaccines). Thus we save many children whose general vigor or immune systems wouldn't have saved them in the past; they must, as a group, create at least slight changes in the human gene pool. In fact, Jonas and Klein may be right in asserting that the children who now survive childhood viral ills have begun to form the nucleus of a new sub-species.

Consider as well children saved from bacterial and pro-tozoan infections, and those preserved from immediate or eventual death caused by physical and mental defects. Add the effects of exposure to X-rays, radiation, synthetic hormones, mood-altering drugs, and literally a million other synthetic compounds that have been entering the air, earth, and water. Add the inspired or inept efforts of genetic engineers, acting in increasing numbers on species from yeasts and bacteria to humans. Add the behavioral effects of these physical changes. A new subspecies of humans probably is being created, and we cannot guess what it will be like. Perhaps weaker, diseased, and ridden wth destructive traits. Perhaps gifted with new brilliance and cooperative, nurturing capacities. Perhaps both. Perhaps, like Jonas's and Klein's debilitated simians, about to perform some unpredictable turn of adaptation, drawing on great strengths and resilience on which to survive and thrive.

This view is not apocalyptic; it does not denigrate the human past or future. It does refuse to put humans alone at the center of the universe, exempt from the forces that affect all other creatures. The attitude is warranted, considering that biocataclysms have struck the world's entire living population often in historic times alone.

Those who think viral epidemic and regressive evolution too much of a bad thing should look at some new and increasingly popular theories about far grander disasters. One explains the extinction of the dinosaurs, which allowed the tiny, early mammals to inherit the earth.

Some sixty-five million years ago, up to three-quarters of the earth's species — the land dinosaurs, great marine reptiles, flying reptiles, and a vast number of tiny marine creatures that form the base of the marine food chain — all vanished. It is a biocataclysm worth pondering for its human implications.

This cataclysm is called the Cretaceous-Tertiary boundary event, a portentous name that befits a literally earth-shaking occurrence. It has long been depicted as a gradual climatic change to which cold-blooded animals could not adapt; textbooks, children's books, and the film *Fantasia* have left in millions of minds a picture of dinosaurs gasping and dying in hot dust. Again, the picture is one of orderly change in which higher, more complex species succeeded through a gradual process.

Only some half-dozen years ago, a quite different explanation began to take shape. It was far more dramatic, and that itself made some people doubt it. But the research of a father-son team of scientists from the University of California at Berkeley made a geological discovery in Italy that had stunning implications about the end of the age of the dinosaurs.

Physicist Luis Alvarez and his geologist son, Walter Alvarez, looked in the field and in the laboratory at the geological stratum that lay between the Cretaceous period of the dinosaurs and the Tertiary period that succeeded it. Other scientists had noticed before them that since it was very thin, it represented a very short period of time. Actually, it was so thin that it could hardly represent a gradual change in world climate and vegetation. In the laboratory, using the most advanced methods of analysis, the Alvarezes found that the layer contained an astonishing excess of iridium, a rare metal related to platinum.

Only tiny amounts of iridium exist in the earth's crust; scientists think that most of this planet's iridium settled long ago in its molten core. There is only one other place such concentrations of iridium could come from, and that is meteorites. The implications of the Alvarez discovery sent other researchers testing the Cretaceous-Tertiary boundary for iridium all over the world, from Denmark to New Zealand to the world's ocean beds. They kept finding great excesses of iridium and of osmium, another rare metal related to platinum and far commoner in meteorites than on earth. They also kept finding tektites, the glassy material created when a meteor's impact sends debris flying off to cool in new form and descend as fallout.

A new theory took shape as more evidence came in: The evolution of our entire biosphere changed violently and abruptly when a comet some ten kilometers across landed in one of the oceans. It heated the seas and the atmosphere, released cyanide gas, and left a mass of dust in the stratosphere for years, causing darkness and heat and hindering photosynthesis. It happened quickly; the layer separating the dinosaur age from the age of mammals may represent as little as fifty years in Spain. The impact, says Dr. Kenneth Hsü of Zurich, would have had results that "match quite closely the extinctions observed in the paleontological record." The Alvarezes infer that the earth was struck by one of the larger asteroids whose orbits cross that of earth.

This theory might have lain a while amid heated debate by specialists; however, researchers continued to follow up the implications, and some of them found signs of yet another meteor that wrought cataclysmic changes. There were drillings on the floors of the Caribbean, Indian, and Pacific oceans, Denmark, and Colorado. E. P. Glass, R. Ganapathy, and the Alvarezes discovered a thin layer loaded with iridium at the abrupt end of the Eocene epoch, about thirty-four million years ago. Ganapathy calculates that a meteor three kilometers in diameter, weighing at least fifty billion tons, landed in the Caribbean, left tektites strewn halfway around the world, and created enough environmental fallout to cause a sudden die-off of both land and sea species. Both the Eocene and the Cretaceous-Tertiary events, he said, show strong evidence of wide-spread extinctions, and "the implication that major meteorite impacts have played a role in the evolution of life on earth." People who want to imagine the effects of a "limited" nuclear war might use these cataclysms as measuring sticks.

Not all scientists have leaped eagerly at the theory. Some say the iridium came from volcanic eruptions, others that the chief cause of mass extinctions was cooling of the climate unrelated to meteors. Berkeley paleontologist William Clemens studied fossil dinosaurs in Montana and concluded, as some others had, that an asteroid did almost decimate marine life sixty-five million years ago, but it did not do in the dinosaurs. They had already vanished, he said, when the meteor struck. Walter Alvarez disagrees; he says that the boundary layer in Montana represents ten thousand years at most, a blink of the eye in evolutionary terms — certainly a mere moment considering the millions of years during which dinosaurs dominated the earth.

As this book is about to go to press, the theory takes another leap forward. Scientists at Berkeley, the University of Chicago, and NASA have studied the frequencies of extinctions and of objects colliding with the earth, and they find a regularity that they think can be explained only by an astral body's orbit. Two pairs of researchers now say that the sun has a companion star they call Nemesis, which sends comets hurtling toward the earth every twenty-eight million years, causing mass extinctions. The star has not been seen, but calculations suggest that it exists and is due to visit us again in'fourteen million years.

Disagreement continues, and much remains to be learned. Many scientists agree with the Alvarezes and their colleagues that the iridium marker has evolutionary importance and will help determine time sequences in digs all over the world. Scientist Erle Kauffman considers it most significant that his colleagues are willing to consider views other than the traditional gradualism: "It is a great philosophical breakthrough for geologists to accept catastrophe as a normal part of Earth history."

Some claim that dinosaurs and asteroids have nothing to do with each other. The answers are important not only for learning the facts and understanding evolution better, but for shaping attitudes toward biological processes in all species, including man. This is quite clear when one considers a theory put forward recently by Paul Martin of the University of Arizona, about the disappearance of some fifty-five species of large animals ten thousand years ago, at the end of the last glacial period. Because the mastodon, mammoth, giant ground sloth, and saber-tooth tiger disappeared when the glaciers retreated, many people assumed that the climatic and other environmental results caused the extinctions. Martin believes that the reason was hunting by humans; he puts the extinctions at the same date as the start of human occupation in parts of the New World. He also points out that the species disappeared much more rapidly than the climate changed. To those who doubt overhunting could cause the extinctions, he refers to the example of Madagascar, first settled by humans only a thousand years ago, with the prompt disappearance of many large animals.

I am not competent to judge in the disputes about whether an asteroid killed off the dinosaurs and whether hunters wiped out the saber-tooth tiger. Neither can I judge whether the theory of regressive evolution excels competing theories; however, the idea may now seem less eccentric than it did at first glance. Which side even specialists take may depend as much on temperament and frame of mind as on fact. I myself am wary of apocryphal thinking and disaster scenarios, and the complex interplay of biosphere and environment so fascinates me that I would rather contemplate it than seek a "big bang" theory. Some people love such simplification, its violence and finality. Despite myself, I must hesitate with respectful curiosity before certain cataclysmic theories.

There is no doubt that meteors have struck the earth, and that epidemics have ravaged it. The biohistory of humans and their world has not been an unbroken series of steps for the better. It has included disaster and triumph over disaster, often in ways we cannot yet understand. New conquests in biohistory will rise not only from new laboratory instruments and observations but from the flexibility that allows continuing change and broadening of one's views.

Biohistory has a future; all history does. History is more than accumulated information, more even than informed interpretation. It is the way we continually reinterpret events to satisfy our changing preoccupations, and restate our sense of ourselves and the world we live in. Thus each generation repaints the portrait of its past, keeps seeking a new present, and revises its expectations of the future. In short, history is a changing state of mind.

Biohistory is a quite special state of mind, very different from that of traditional history and natural science. It is distinguished by a wide-ranging view of what have been thought distinct parts of life and of scholarship; it flourishes through a synthesizing imagination. When it looks at Napoleon or Poe, it takes into account not only politics and literature but those men's emotional histories as best understood by psychiatry today, their physical histories as best seen by modern medicine, and the interaction of mind and body in a social context. Looking at the cultural past, biohistory looks at behavior and feelings inherited from our evolutionary ancestors and at environmental influences. Viewing humans' physical remains, it tries to infer their culture, their daily lives, their feelings and beliefs. Biohistory studies not only the effects of disease on culture but the effects of culture on disease. Regarding the human species, it considers the entire biosphere, from trace metals in the air to the ringing of biological clocks in our emotions.

This book has shown just a handful of ventures in biohistory; there are dozens of others I would have liked to pursue. Some are studies of individuals. Since Goya suffered what was known as the painter's disease, I would like to see how much it affected other great painters. Some scientists have suggested a related case worth following up, that of Sir Isaac Newton, whose life may have been changed drastically by a bout of severe physical and mental illness that could well have resulted from similar heavy-metal poisoning — swallowing and inhaling the mercury he used so extensively in his laboratory experiments. His diaries suggest that this happened, and one must recall that the use of mercury in making felt for hats was responsible for the phrase "mad as a hatter." There is also a good biohistorical study to be made of Alexander the Great, who has variously been called an alcoholic, epileptic, and victim of "the malady of power."

Many families and small populations could be subjects of interesting studies. The hemophiliac Romanov dynasty has already received a good bit of attention; our knowledge of genetically determined diseases has grown so much in recent years that major new studies should probably be done of many ruling lines from ancient Egypt to modern Europe. Fascinating studies could also be done of highly inbred small populations, from Paleolithic-level groups in Borneo to small communities in the Ozarks and the northeastern U.S.

Studies of large populations can now be done in promising new ways. A full biohistory of malaria and its impact on world civilization could occupy one person's entire life. Malaria's relationship with sickle-cell anemia (which confers some protection against malaria) has deeply affected African and Afro-American history. The subject has been written about much in recent years, but the disease's full impact on ancient and modern societies remains to be fully portrayed. Studies of hemoglobin, blood types, and tissue typing may soon allow us to trace population shifts where no written records existed. The results could be correlated with malaria maps.

Quite different studies are possible as well. For decades, psychiatrists and anthropologists have tried to relate child-rearing to cultural patterns. A definitive study of the psychosocial impact of wet-nursing and bottle-feeding, for instance, remains to be done, drawing not only the usual disciplines but on modern research on mother-infant bonding.

Biohistory also suggests that much can still be learned about the sense of smell as a force in human evolution, behavior, and relationships. Cross-cultural studies will have to be correlated with social and psychological observations. Then we will know if some biologists are right in suggesting that whether we like what others think or do may be less important than whether we like the way they smell.

Two studies particularly nag at me. One is the effect on humanity of the first long-distance weapons, which we examined in chapter 5. We say that nuclear arms have changed human life forever, and that is true. But perhaps as big or bigger was the influence of the first spear, sling, or bow and arrow — whatever first allowed killing at a distance. It takes courage, cunning, strength, and lots of hatred to kill another person with one's bare hands or even with a rock or stick. Imagine the terror, exultation, and awe of the first person able to kill from afar, without touching, without having to see the other person as an individual. Perhaps the weapon was first invented for hunting, but the implication of its first use on another person must have been staggering. It must have seemed that the extinction of humanity, as anyone could then conceive it, became a possibility.

Like other social, aggressive creatures, humans have not only a great potential for violence but strong ways to control and appease violence. All of that is built genetically into the operations of the midbrain, a seat of feeling more than of logic. The growing cerebral cortex, the reasoning part of the brain, developed technology, including the technology of weapons. Long-distance killing and the remorseless cortex made humans the first and only super-killers on earth, deadly to other species and to themselves. We need to better understand this gulf between the reasoning and feeling parts of the brain.

Another subject that seems to me to cry for special study is how boys become men and how girls become women. The question is so big that one must seize one corner of it and use it as a handle. We have begun to learn something about how men act in groups; we must learn more about how early relationships and boys' play prepares them. There is now some compelling research on the antecedents of male group and social behavior in the observation of other social species. Only a decade ago, Tiger and Shepher produced a study of enormous importance on how women function in groups, called *Women on the Kibbutz*. Interest is high in women's thinking, feeling, and behavior. The time is ready not only for advocacy for women's rights but for more knowledge of a subject badly ignored. For the sake of women, men, and children, we need as much study of women as of men, and tools for such study are better than ever.

I hope that others will pursue these ventures. There is one I am saving for myself. Some day I hope to write the biohistory of my family. My distant ancestors probably roved as nomadic shepherds or rode camels about the Near East. Somehow my father's family ended up a century and a half ago around Minsk, in Russia; my mother's family ended up in Ukrainia, around Odessa and Kiev. They survived those ghastly hostilities in which people treat members of other ethnic groups as other species. They survived by forming large, loyal clans. Both families came to the United States and entered a new course of social and biological history, including extensive intermarriage with other peoples. They have had a genetic, medical, and social history, and also that sort of history peculiar to families. Should I write that history, it will do what all biohistory must directly or indirectly do. It will bring history home.

Bibliography

$\mathcal{P}$EOPLE often ignore bibliographies; often they are right. This one is meant to be used, not to lie like a toppled tombstone at the back of the book. As readers, we all want authors to throw us a rope. Here is a short one.

A complete scholarly bibliography on any chapter in this book could be a volume in itself. For instance, several hundred thousand items have appeared in print about Napoleon. Furthermore, some of the sources used for this book are specialized; as the old joke about penguins has it, they would interest only another penguin. My purpose here is twofold, to list most works extensively quoted or drawn on and to give readers a springboard for pursuing these ventures in biohistory. Books are also recommended for each chapter that provide detailed, scholarly bibliographies.

This author believes in going out on a limb and saying which sources he considers good, mediocre, or bunk. It is an attempt to save readers time and bother. Asterisks mark works that are especially important or readable. There are also indications, when needed, of which works

are for general readers and which for scholars or people
with special backgrounds.

Chapter 1: Napoleon's Glands

There are entire periodicals devoted to listing publications about
Napoleon, and the literature is extensive in several languages.
Butterfield's short book is a brief, readable introduction. The general
reader can get Felix Markham's book in paperback and use his
bibliography as an initial guide. This chapter has drawn on the firsthand
accounts of Napoleon's years at St. Helena by those who knew him
there — Antommarchi, Bertrand, de las Cases, Gourgaud, Marchand,
Montholon, and others. These writers are quoted plentifully in most
extensive works on Napoleon's last years. Among the respected general
works on Napoleon's life are those by Fournier, Rose, and Thompson.
Much of the old medical literature, and even some of the new, is purely
for scholars or good only as intellectual camp, but is listed because it
is quoted or discussed. Adler is quoted by Way. Yvan, Carnot, and
Dunlop are quoted by Richardson. Abbatucci is quoted by Brice.

*Altick, Richard. *Lives and Letters*. New York: 1966. About literary
    biography, but gives a good, thoughtful overview of the nature
    and problems of biography writing.
Antommarchi, Francesco. *The Last Days of Napoleon*. London: 1826.
Arnott, A. *An Account of the Last Illness, Decease, and Post-Mortem
    Appearance of Napoleon Bonaparte*. London: 1822.
Aubry, O. *St. Helena*. London: 1937.
Ayer, Wardner. "Napoleon Buonaparte and Schistosomiasis or Bil-
    harziasis." *New York State Journal of Medicine* 66 (1966): 2295–
    2301. Interesting, thorough, convincing.
Bertrand, Henri-Gratien. *Napoleon at St. Helena*. London: 1953.
Brice, Raoul. *The Riddle of Napoleon*. London: 1937. Eccentric.
*Butterfield, Herbert. *Napoleon*. New York: 1956. An excellent and
    quite readable short introduction to Napoleon and his impact on
    Europe. Good for those starting from scratch on the subject.
Cabanes, A. *Curious Bypaths of History*. Paris: 1898. Curiosa.
*Cartwright, Frederick. *Disease and History*. New York: 1972. One of
    the best popular books on disease and epidemics as biohistory.
    Although some details are already slightly dated, this book remains
    informative and entertaining.
Chaplin, Arnold. *The Illness and Death of Napoleon Bonaparte*. Lon-
    don: 1913.

Clark, L. Pierce. "The Narcissism of Napoleon," *Medical Journal and Record* (1929): 442 ff. and 521 ff.

Cobb, Ivo. *The Glands of Destiny: A Study of Personality.* London: 1927. Glands of what?

Desmond, Shaw. *Personality and Power.* London: 1950. Interesting but sometimes overambitious speculation.

Fisher, H. A. L. *Napoleon Bonaparte.* Oxford: 1912. Good short biography.

Forschufvud, Sten. *Who Killed Napoleon?* London: 1962. The arsenic theory.

*Fournier, August. *Napoleon: A Biography.* London: 1911. One of the great, authoritative biographies, written a century ago by a German scholar.

Ganière, Paul. *Napoleon at Sainte-Hélène.* Paris: 1960. Useful.

Gourgaud, Gaspar. *Journal de Saint-Hélène.* Paris: 1899.

Guthrie, Leonard. "Did Napoleon Suffer from Hypopituitarism?" *Lancet* 11 (1913): 623.

Henry, Walter. *Events of a Military Life.* London: 1843.

Hillemand, Pierre. *Pathologie de Napoleon.* Paris: 1970.

Jonas, David, and Jonas, Doris. *Sex & Status.* New York: 1975. An interesting book by a psychiatrist and an anthropologist on the psychology and biology of sex and power. Indirectly but significantly bears on Napoleon.

Kemble, J. *Napoleon Immortal.* New York: 1959. Useful. Reviews much French medical literature. Supports the Fröhlich syndrome theory.

Korngold, Ralph. *The Last Years of Napoleon.* New York: 1959. Important source with a useful bibliography.

Las Cases, Comte de. *Memorial de Ste Hélène.* Paris: 1823.

L'Estaing, Hugh. *The Pathology of Leadership.* New York: 1970. A thoughtful, provocative work on the so-called disease of power; worth reading, sometimes even to argue with.

Lewin, Peter. "News from the Field." *Paleopathology Newsletter* 36 (1982): 5–6. Arguing with the arsenic theory.

Lewin, Peter, Hancock, R. G., and Voynovich, P. "Napoleon Bonaparte — no evidence of chronic arsenic poisoning." *Nature* 299 (1982): 627–628.

McLaurin, C. *Post Mortem.* New York: 1923. Historical interest only.

Marchand, Louis. *Mémoires de Marchand.* Paris: 1955.

*Markham, Felix. *Napoleon.* New York: 1963. Good biography; not for the browser, yet not highly specialized. The bibliography will get a nonspecialist started on the literature about Napoleon.

Martineau, Gilbert. *La Vie Quotidienne à Saint-Hélène au Temps de Napoléon.* Paris: 1966. About the island in Napoleon's day.

Masson, Frédéric. *Napoleon at St. Helena.* London: 1949.

Montholon, Charles-Tristan. *History of the Captivity of Napoleon at St. Helena.* London: 1846.

Neruda, Pablo. *Memoirs.* New York: 1977.

Ober, William. *Boswell's Clap and Other Essays.* Carbondale, Ill.: 1979 Interesting and fun.

O'Meara, Barry. *Napoleon in Exile.* London: 1822.

Richardson, Frank. *Napoleon: Bisexual Emperor.* New York: 1972. Odd theory, very odd.

Rose, J. Holland. *The Personality of Napoleon.* London: 1912.

———. *The Life of Napoleon.* London: 1934. Two major works by a major biographer.

Sokoloff, Boris. *Napoleon: A Doctor's Biography.* New York: 1937. Hastens where the thoughtful fear to tread, making cases of malaria, tuberculosis, pituitary problems, and more.

Stekel, Wilhelm. *Impotence in the Male.* London: 1953.

*Thompson, J. M. *Napoleon Bonaparte. His Rise and Fall.* London: 1952. Good biography.

Way, Lewis. *Adler's Place in Psychology.* London: 1950.

Weider, Ben, and Hapgood, David. *The Murder of Napoleon.* New York: 1982. Popularizes the arsenic-poisoning theory; dramatic, sometimes melodramatic.

Chapter 2: Goya sans Syphilis

There is no definitive biography of Goya, but many scattered writings in many languages. The big, beautiful, and expensive book by Gassier and Wilson gives one some text and a lot of Goya's major works. Some important writings on lead and lead poisoning are cited below; many are left for the chapter devoted entirely to that subject (including those of Chisholm). Zapater is quoted by Niederland. I want to thank Dr. Niederland for his kind help.

Böhme, Gerhard. *"Die Taubheit des Malers Francisco de Goya."* Zeitschrift für Laryngologie, Rhinologie, Otologie 44 (1965): 443–447.

Canaday, John. "Goya and Horror." *Horizon* 10 (1968): 90.

Cawthorne, Terence. "Goya's Illness." *Proceedings of the Royal Society of Medicine* 55 (1962): 213–217.

Doerner, Max. *The Materials of the Artist and Their Use in Painting.*

New York: 1949. Interesting work for the specialist, recreating Goya's palette.

Ferm, Vergil, and Carpenter, Stanley J. "Developmental Malformations Resulting from the Administration of Lead Salts." *Experimental and Molecular Pathology* 7 (1967): 208–213.

*Gassier, Pierre, and Wilson, Juliet. *The Life and Complete Work of Francisco Goya.* New York: 1971. A massive, handsome volume that contains an adequate brief life of Goya and reproduces his major works in many genres and media.

Gautier, Théophile. *Wanderings in Spain.* London: 1853.

Glendinning, Oliver. *Goya and His Critics.* New Haven: 1977.

Goya, Francisco. *Caprichos.* 2 vols. Princeton: 1953.

Hammond, P. B. "Lead Poisoning: An Old Problem with a New Dimension." In Frank R. Blood, ed., *Essays in Toxicology,* Vol. I, New York: 1969.

Harris, Thomas. *Goya: Engravings and Lithographs.* 2 vols. Oxford: 1964.

Huxley, Aldous. *The Complete Etchings of Goya.* New York: 1943.

*Lewis, D. B. Wyndham. *The World of Goya.* London: 1968. Not a definitive biography, but a lively one. A good start for the nonspecialist.

*Licht, Fred, ed. *Goya in Perspective.* Englewood Cliffs, N.J.: 1973. Good collection of writings on Goya, including excerpts from Baudelaire, Gautier, and Goya commentator Folke Nordström. Useful bibliography, including works in several languages.

Malraux, Andre. *Saturn: An Essay on Goya.* New York: 1957.

*Niederland, William. "Goya's Illness." *New York State Journal of Medicine,* Feb. 1, 1972, pp. 413–418. A beautiful example of biohistorical biography at its best.

———. "Psychoanalytic Approaches to Artistic Creativity." *Psychoanalytic Quarterly* 45 (1976): 185–212.

Nordström, Folke. *Goya, Saturn, and Melancholy: Studies in the Art of Goya.* Stockholm: 1962.

Ramazzini, Bernardino. *Diseases of Workers.* New York: 1964.

Rouanet, G. *Le Mystère Goya.* Paris: 1960.

Schmid, F. "The Technique of Goya." In D. C. Rich, ed., *The Art of Goya.* Chicago: 1941.

Shapiro, S. L. "The Fateful Illness of Francisco Goya." *Eye, Ear, Nose and Throat Monthly* 45 (1966): 89 ff.

Tanquerel des Planches, L. *Traité des Maladies de Plomb ou Saturnines.* Paris: 1839.

*Waldron, H. A., and Stofen, D. *Sub-Clinical Lead Poisoning.* New York: 1974. Excellent technical work.

Zimbardo, P. G., Andersen, S. M., and Kabat, L. G. "Induced

Hearing Deficit Generates Experimental Paranoia." *Science* 212 (1981): 1529–1531.

Chapter 3: What Ailed Poor Poe?

Poe, like Napoleon, has drawn many biographers and commentators he didn't deserve. There are books and periodicals of bibliography alone. Today all serious study of Poe should start with Quinn's book; for a less exhaustive approach, try Wagenknecht. Altogether, writings on Poe from a medical and psychological standpoint offer a lot of strange junk. Praz gives good background, Carlson's and Regan's collections a good critical introduction. For the present, the "Virginia edition" of Poe's work in seventeen volumes remains the standard but still not definitive edition of Poe's work. There are enough adequate paperback collections for any reader but a Poe scholar to easily find a good sampling and most of the major works. Burr and Graham are quoted by Quinn; Gilfillan and Lowell by Regan; Eliot, James, Shaw, and Willis by Carlson. I want to thank Dr. Timothy Perper and Martha Cornog Perper for their help in researching alcohol dehydrogenase.

Allen, Hervey. *Israfel: The Life and Times of Edgar Allan Poe.* New York: 1934. A popular and lively biography of Poe, somewhat romanticized and reckless. Try Wagenknecht instead.

Allen, Michael. *Poe and the British Magazine Tradition.* New York: 1969. Shows in detail the roots of Poe's work in events and styles of his time, making it seem less idiosyncratic.

Baudelaire, Charles. *Fatal Destinies: The Edgar Allan Poe Essays.* Woodhaven, N.Y.: 1981. A handy translation of Baudelaire's essays on Poe.

Bonaparte, Marie. *The Life and Works of Edgar Allan Poe: A Psycho-Analytic Interpretation.* London: 1949. Literary psychoanalysis at its worst.

Campbell, Killis. *The Mind of Poe and Other Studies.* Cambridge, Mass.: 1933.

*Carlson, Eric W., ed. *The Recognition of Edgar Allan Poe.* Ann Arbor: 1970. A paperback collection of writings on Poe from contemporaries such as Nathaniel Willis to Baudelaire and Dostoevski, and on to Mallarmé, Walt Whitman, G. B. Shaw, D. H. Lawrence, and T. S. Eliot. A very handy compilation for someone dipping into Poe criticism.

Ewing, John, et al. "Alcohol Sensitivity and Ethnic Background." *American Journal of Psychiatry* 131 (1974): 206–210.

Hyneman, Esther. *Edgar Allen Poe: An Annotated Bibliography.*

Boston: 1974. Covers the period 1827–1973. Can be supplemented with the periodical called *Poe Newsletter* and then *Poe Studies* for the years 1968–1978.

Krutch, Joseph Wood. *Edgar Allan Poe: A Study in Genius*. New York: 1926. A curiosity, outstanding for its venom.

Marks, Jeannette. *Genius and Disaster: Studies in Drugs and Genius*. New York: 1925. Almost as bad as Bonaparte and Krutch.

Maudsley, Henry. "Edgar Allan Poe." *American Journal of Insanity* 18 (Oct. 1850): 167.

Miller, Perry. *The Raven and the Whale*. New York: 1956.

Pickering, George. *Creative Malady*. New York: 1974. Interesting exploration of physical illness in great nineteenth-century creative figures. Without treating Poe, suggests interesting ideas about health, sickness, and creativity.

Poe, Edgar Allan. *The Works of the Late Edgar Allan Poe: With Notices of His Life and Genius*. New York: 1850. The edition with the historic Griswold libels.

———. *The Complete Works*. 17 vols. New York: 1902. Until supplanted, the standard edition. A better edition has long been in preparation by Harvard University Press; three volumes have so far appeared, the poems (1969) and the tales and sketches (2 vols., 1978).

———. *Letters*. 2 vols. Cambridge, Mass.: 1949. Standard edition.

———. *Poems*. Charlottesville: 1965. Standard edition.

*Praz, Mario. *The Romantic Agony*. New York: 1956. A classic of literary scholarship, about the themes of literature throughout the Western world in Poe's era.

*Quinn, Arthur Hobson. *Edgar Allan Poe: A Critical Biography*. New York: 1941. The classic Poe biography, and a model of scholarship. A must for anyone interested in dipping more than shallowly into Poe.

Regan, Robert, ed. *Poe: A Collection of Critical Essays*. Englewood Cliffs, N.J.: 1967. Handy compilation.

Robertson, John W. *Edgar Allan Poe: A Psychopathic Study*. New York: 1923.

Seto, Anthony, et al. "Biochemical Correlates of Ethanol-Induced Flushing in Orientals." *Journal of Studies on Alcohol* 39 (1978): 1–11.

Stamatoyannopoulos, George; Chen, Shi-Han; and Fukui, Miyoshi. "Liver Alcohol Dehydrogenase in Japanese." *American Journal of Human Genetics* 27 (1975): 789–796.

*Wagenknecht, Edward. *Edgar Allan Poe: The Man Behind the Legend*. New York: 1963. A lively and accurate biography for those who don't want to take on Quinn's exhaustive volume.

Wolff, Peter. "Vasomotor Sensivitity to Alcohol in Diverse Mongoloid Populations." *American Journal of Human Genetics* 25 (1973): 193–199.

Woodberry, George. *The Life of Edgar Allan Poe.* 2 vols. Boston: 1909. The major biography until Quinn's appeared; dated but useful to specialists.

Yoshida, Akira; Impraim, Chaka; and Huang, I-Yih. "Enzymatic and Structural Differences between Usual and Atypical Human Liver Alcohol Dehydrogenases." *The Journal of Biological Chemistry* 256 (1981): 12430–12436.

Young, Philip. "The Earlier Psychologists and Poe." *American Literature* 27 (1950): 442–454. A good early attempt to understand what early psychologists had and hadn't made of Poe.

Zilboorg, Gregory. *A History of Medical Psychology.* New York: 1941. Still unsurpassed as background for people interested in the history of psychology. Strongly recommended to those who are more than visiting the subject.

Chapter 4: Mummy Powder, Mummy Blood

The book edited by Aidan and Eve Cockburn puts together in one volume everything one wants to know about mummies, from their history and geographical distribution about the world to laboratory analysis techniques. It is written for the scientist but may interest the ambitious layman with some medical background. The Brothwell and Sandison book, though a bit dated, is also useful, and also for specialists. Laymen will enjoy the book on bog mummies by Glob. My thanks to Dr. Michael Zimmerman for his suggestions and review of this chapter.

*Brothwell, Don, and Sandison, A. T., eds. *Diseases in Antiquity.* Springfield, Ill.: 1967. Although a bit dated, a must for people seriously interested in diseases in ancient peoples. It contains many landmark papers, including a good one on pseudopathology by biohistorian Calvin Wells. For specialists or those developing a technical interest.

Cockburn, Aidan. *The Evolution and Eradication of Infectious Diseases.* Baltimore: 1963. One of the important books of recent decades on the history of diseases.

———. "Paleopathology and Its Association." *Journal of the American Medical Association* 240 (1978): 151–153.

*Cockburn, Aidan, and Cockburn, Eve, eds. *Mummies, Disease, and*

Ancient Cultures. Cambridge, England: 1980. The book lives up to its ambitious title; it is *the* comprehensive and indispensable compendium on the subject. Includes essays on mummies from Peru to Japan, on the mummies PUM II, Rom I, and Nakht, on dental health in ancient Egypt. Each chapter has its own bibliography. Deals with laboratory methods from blood-typing to electron microscopy.

*Glob, P. V. *The Bog People*. New York: 1971. A readable popular book by the outstanding Danish researcher on bog mummies.

Harris, H. A. *Bone Growth in Health and Disease*. London: 1933. The landmark work on "Harris lines."

Harris, James, and Weeks, Kent. *X-Raying the Pharaohs*. New York: 1973. For laymen, with many photographs. Very interesting introduction to the modern study of mummies. See below, Harris and Wente.

Harris, James, and Wente, Edward. *An X-Ray Atlas of the Royal Mummies*. Chicago: 1980. For specialists. A major work, from the research on which the popular book of Harris and Weeks (see above) developed.

Harrison, R. G., and Connolly, R. C. "Kinship of Smenkhare and Tutankamon Demonstrated Serologically." *Nature* 224 (1969): 325–326.

Kleiss, Ekkehard. "Some Examples of Natural Mummies." *Paleopathology Newsletter* No. 20 (1977): 5–6.

Lekk, F. Filce. "Paleodontology of the Nile Valley." *Paleopathology Newsletter* No. 33 (1981): 9–12.

Pettigrew, Thomas. *The History of Egyptian Mummies*. London: 1834.

Ruffer, Marc A. "Notes on the Presence of 'Bilharzia Haematoria' in Egyptian Mummies of the Twentieth Dynasty (1250–1000 B.C.)." In Brothwell and Sandison, eds., see above. A landmark paper.

Shimken, M. D. "Some Historical Landmarks in Cancer Epidemiology." In D. Schottenfeld, ed., *Cancer Epidemiology and Prevention: Current Concepts*. Springfield, Ill.: 1975, pp. 60–74.

Stasny, P. "HL-A Antigens in Mummified PreColumbian Tissues." *Science* 183 (1974): 864–866.

Steinbock, R. Ted. *Paleopathological Diagnosis and Interpretation*. Springfield, Ill.: 1976. Excellent technical work on ancient bone pathology. Extensive bibliography.

Wei, O. "Internal Organs of 2100 Year Old Female Corpse." *Lancet* 2 (1973): 1198.

Zimmerman, Michael. "Paleopathological Diagnosis Based on Experimental Mummification." *American Journal of Physical Anthropology* 51 (1973): 235–253.

————. "An Experimental Study of Mummification Pertinent to the Antiquity of Cancer." *Cancer* 40 (1977): 1358–1362.

Chapter 5: Dry Bones

More than any other chapter, this one draws on numerous scattered and specialized scientific papers, sometimes a half dozen bearing on one small point. I have listed many of those quoted directly or indirectly, some that are landmarks in the field. No work exists, to my knowledge, to introduce laymen to this fascinating field. I have drawn heavily on the invaluable *Paleopathology Newsletter*. The book of Brothwell and Sandison, though now somewhat dated, is still indispenable; the Cockburns' book on mummies, cited for the previous chapter, is an equally valuable update. Steinbock's book, for specialists, has exhaustive bibliographies.

Angel, J. L. "Patterns of Fractures from Neolithic to Modern Times." *Anthrop. Kozlemenyek* 18 (1974): 9–18. Summary in *Paleopathology Newsletter* 12 (1975): 15.

————. "Osteoarthritis in Prehistoric Turkey and Medieval Byzantium." *Henry Ford Hospital Medical Journal* 27 (1979): 38–43. This issue of the journal consists of "Paleopathology Association Monograph No. 3," a very useful collection of papers.

Benfer, Robert, et al. "Adaptations to Sedentism and Food Production: The Paloma Project." *Paleopathology Newsletter* 37 (1982): 6–8.

————. Idem. *Paleopathology Newsletter* 36 (1981): 11–13.

*Brothwell, Don, and Sandison, A. T., eds. *Diseases in Antiquity.* Springfield, Ill.: 1967. As described in bibliography for chapter 4, indispensable.

Bryant, Vaughn, Jr., and Williams-Dena, Glenna. "The Coprolites of Man." *Scientific American* 232 (Jan. 1975): 100–109. Somewhat dated, but useful for laymen.

Clarke, Steven. "Mortality Trends in Prehistoric Populations." *Human Biology* 49 (1977): 181–186.

*Cockburn, Aidan, and Cockburn, Eve, eds. *Mummies, Disease, and Ancient Cultures.* Cambridge, England: 1980. As described in bibliography for chapter 4, indispensable.

Cockburn, Aidan; Duncan, Howard; and Riddle, Jeanne. "Arthritis, Ancient and Modern." *Henry Ford Hospital Medical Journal* 27 (1979): 74–79.

"Data Indicate Neanderthal Man Used Herbs for Healing 60,000 Years Ago." *The New York Times*, August 26, 1975.

Ferguson, Mark. "Cleft Palate Past and Present." *Paleopathology Newsletter* 24 (1978): 5–8.
Gregg, John. "News from the Field." *Paleopathology Newsletter* 24 (1978): 4, 18. On the Crow Creek massacre.
Hatch, J. W., and Geidel, R. A. "Tracing Status and Diet in Prehistoric Tennessee." *Archaeology* 36 (1983): 56–59.
Hooton, Earnest. *The Indians of Pecos Pueblo.* New Haven: 1930.
Korfmann, Manfred. "The Sling as a Weapon." *Scientific American* 229 (October 1973): 34–42.
Lallo, J. W., and Rose, J. C. "Patterns of Stress, Disease, and Mortality in Two Prehistoric Populations from North America." *Journal of Human Evolution* 8 (1979): 323–335.
Leisen, James, and Duncan, Howard. "The Impact of Rheumatic Disease on Society." *Henry Ford Hospital Medical Journal* 27 (1979): 70–73.
Lewin, Roger. "Protohuman Activity Etched in Fossil Bones." *Science* 213 (1981): 123–124.
———. "Isotopes Give Clues to Past Diets." *Science* 220 (1983): 1369.
Lovejoy, C. O., and Heiple, K. G. "The Analysis of Fractures in Skeletal Populations." *American Journal of Physical Anthropology* 55 (1981): 529–541.
Loy, Thomas. "Prehistoric Blood Residues: Detection on Tool Surfaces and Identification of Species of Origin." *Science* 220 (1983): 1269–1270.
Macadam, Patty Stuart. "A Small Skeletal Sample from Northern Ghana." *Paleopathology Newsletter* 33 (1981): 5–7.
McHenry, Henry, and Schultz, Peter. "The Association between Harris Lines and Enamel Hypoplasia in Prehistoric California Indians." *American Journal of Physical Anthropology* 44 (1976): 507–512.
Moore, P. D., and Webb, J. A. *An Illustrated Guide to Pollen Analysis.* New York: 1979.
"New Dig Unearths the Pathos of Vesuvius." *The New York Times,* November 17, 1982.
Pickering, Robert. "Hunter-Gatherer/Agriculturalist Arthritic Patterns: A Preliminary Investigation." *Henry Ford Hospital Medical Journal* 27 (1979): 50–53.
Redman, C. L., et al., eds. *Social Archaeology: Beyond Subsistence and Dating.* New York: 1978.
"Research Yields Surprises about Early Human Diets." *The New York Times,* May 15, 1979.
Saul, F. "Disease in the Maya Area." In T. P. Culbert, ed., *The Classic Maya Collapse.* Albuquerque: 1973.
*Steinbock, R. Ted. *Paleopathological Diagnosis and Interpretation.*

Springfield, Ill.: 1976. Essential for knowing the scientific literature. Extensive bibliographies.

Straus, Lawrence G., et al. "Ice-Age Subsistence in Northern Spain." *Scientific American* 242 (June 1980): 142–152.

Trinkaus, Erik. *The Shanidar Neandertals.* New York: 1983.

Trinkaus, Erik, and Zimmerman, Michael. "Trauma Among the Shanidar Neandertals." *American Journal of Physical Anthropology* 57 (1982): 61–76.

Wells, Calvin. "A New Approach to Paleopathology: Harris Lines." In Brothwell and Sandison, eds., op. cit.

*Wilson, Edward O. *Sociobiology.* Cambridge, Mass.: 1980. An abridged version of a debated but very important work, accessible to the ambitious layman.

Zimmerman, Michael, et al. "Trauma and Trephination in a Peruvian Mummy." *American Journal of Physical Anthropology* 55 (1981): 497–501.

Chapter 6: Biocataclysm

There are now several good books, from introductions for laymen to quite sophisticated and scholarly overviews, of the history of diseases and epidemics. Perhaps the best recent work is that of McNeill, *Plagues and People,* for the serious nonspecialist. Sigerist is dated but still interesting in places. Cartwright's is probably the best recent popular work. Rosebury's book on venereal infections is excellent, as is Gottfried's on the plague. My thanks to Professor Stanley Weinstein for the term biocataclysm.

"AIDS Cases Seen Doubling This Year in San Francisco." *The Wall Street Journal,* March 8, 1984.

Aronson, S. M. "Lead and the Demon Rum in Colonial America." *Rhode Island Medical Journal* 66 (1983): 37–40.

Biraben, J.-N. *Les Hommes et la Peste.* 2 vols. The Hague: 1975. One of the definitive studies of the plague, for serious readers.

Boccaccio, Giovanni. *The Decameron.* London: 1972.

Bowsky, William, ed. *The Black Death: A Turning Point in History?* New York: 1971. Useful collection of excerpts representing several views of the plague and its results.

Burgerdorf, Willy, et al. "Lyme Disease — A Tick-Borne Spirochetosis?" *Science* 216 (1982): 1317–1319.

*Burnet, Macfarlane, and White, David. *Natural History of Infectious Diseases.* Cambridge, England: 1972. 4th ed. After McNeill's (see below), the best wide-ranging book of its kind. Can be read by the ambitious nonspecialist.

*Cartwright, Frank. *Disease and History.* New York: 1972. An engaging introduction for general readers.

Chambers, J. D. *Population, Plague, and Society in Pre-Industrial England.* Oxford: 1972.

Cockburn, Aidan. *The Evolution and Eradication of Infectious Diseases.* Baltimore: 1963. An important book.

Defoe, Daniel. *A Journal of the Plague Year.* New York: 1960. If you've never read it, do yourself a favor.

Dixon, Bernard. *Magnificent Microbes.* New York: 1976. For laymen, on microbes helpful to humans.

Dols, Michael. *The Black Death in the Middle East.* Princeton: 1977.

Fiennes, Richard. *Zoonoses of Primates.* Ithaca: 1967.

Fracastor, Girolamo. *Contagion.* New York: 1930.

Fraser, D. S., and McDade, J. E. "Legionellosis." *Scientific American* 241 (October 1979): 82–83, 186.

Fuller, John G. *Fever! The Hunt for a New Killer Virus.* New York: 1974. On Lassa fever.

Goff, C. W. "Syphilis." In Brothwell, Don, and Sandison, A. T., eds., *Diseases in Antiquity.* Springfield, Ill.: 1967, pp. 279–294.

*Gottfried, Robert. *The Black Death.* New York: 1983. A first-rate biohistory of the plague, its social and environmental context, and its effects. Excellent bibliography. Useful to anyone not a true specialist, and written in clear if not engaging prose.

Gravell, Maneth, et al. "Transmission of Simian Acquired Immunodeficiency Syndrome (SAIDS) with Blood or Filtered Plasma." *Science* 223 (1984): 74–75.

Hackett, C. J. "The Human Treponematoses." In Brothwell, Don, and Sandison, A. T., eds., *Diseases in Antiquity.* Springfield, Ill.: 1967, pp. 152–169. One of the best papers by a major theoretician of the history and evolution of syphilis.

Hohenheim, Theophrastus Von. *Four Treatises of Theophrastus Von Hohenheim, Called Paracelsus.* Baltimore: 1941.

Hudson, E. H. "Treponematosis and Man's Social Evolution." *American Anthropology* 67 (1965): 885–891. A major paper that, like Hackett's (above), is crucial to understanding spirochete infections.

———. "Historical Approach to the Terminology of Syphilis." *Archives of Dermatology* 84 (1961): 546–562.

Laver, W. G. *The Origin of Pandemic Influenza Viruses.* New York: 1983.

*McNeill, William H. *Plagues and People.* New York: 1977. Probably the best single book on disease, history, and culture. At times heavy going for the casual reader, but a must for interested people at all levels of knowledge. Exhaustively referenced.

————. *The Human Condition: An Ecological and Historical View.* Princeton: 1980. Another fine, thoughtful book.

Marx, Jean. "Acquired Immune Deficiency Abroad." *Science* 222 (1983): 998–999.

Procopius. *History of the Wars,* I. New York: 1914.

*Rosebury, Theodor. *Microbes and Morals.* New York: 1973. A fine and well-written biological and social history of sexually transmitted diseases.

Sigerist, Henry. *Civilization and Disease.* Chicago: 1943. Now dated, and brave in its generalizations; one of the first widely read books in the U.S. on the impact of disease on culture. Still worth a look.

Thucydides. *The Peloponnesian War.* London: 1972.

Wilcox, R. R. "Venereal Disease in the Bible." *British Journal of Venereal Disease* 25 (1949): 28–33.

Zinsser, Hans. *Rats, Lice and History.* Boston: 1935. Dated but readable.

Chapter 7: Global Poison

Much of the literature on lead poisoning is highly technical. Waldron, Schroeder, Patterson, and Needleman are among the better-known researchers in the field; the books of Waldron, Needleman, and Lynam et al. are especially useful. A good popular book on the subject waits to be written.

Aub, J. C., et al. *Lead Poisoning.* Baltimore: 1926. Dated; important in its time.

Barltrop, D. "The Prevalence of Pica." *American Journal of Diseases of Children* 112 (1966): 116–123.

Beattie, A. D., et al. "Role of Chronic Low-Level Lead Exposure in the Aetiology of Mental Retardation." *Lancet* No. 7907 (1975): 589–591.

"A Belgian City and Its Poison Air." *New York Post,* October 16, 1974.

Catton, M. J., et al. "Sub-Clinical Neuropathy in Lead Workers." *British Medical Journal* 2 (1970): 80.

Chisholm, J. Julian, Jr. "Lead Poisoning." *Scientific American* 224 (1971): 15–23. Though dated, still the best short overview for laymen I have seen, by a leading researcher.

Chisholm, J. Julian, Jr., and Kaplan, Eugene. "Lead Poisoning in Childhood — Comprehensive Mangement and Prevention." *The Journal of Pediatrics* 73 (1968): 942–950.

"El Paso Smelter Still Poses Lead-Poisoning Peril to Children in Juarez." *The New York Times,* November 28, 1977.

Emmerson, B. T. "Chronic Lead Neuropathy." *Australian Annals of Medicine* 12 (1963): 310.

"EPA Eyes Rule to Phase Out Leaded Gasoline Use." *Oil & Gas Journal* 10 (March 5, 1984): 60.

Ericson, J. E., Skirahata, M. S., and Patterson, C. C. "Skeletal Concentrations of Lead in Ancient Peruvians." *New England Journal of Medicine* 300 (1979): 946–951.

Esposito, John. *Vanishing Air.* New York: 1970. A Ralph Nader Group report on air pollution, including the use of TEL.

Ferm, Vergil, and Carpenter, Stanley J. "Developmental Malformations Resulting from the Administrations of Lead Salts." *Experimental and Molecular Pathology* 7 (1967): 208–213.

Gilfillan, S. C. "Lead Poisoning and the Fall of Rome." *Journal of Occupational Medicine* 1 (1965): 53–60.

Hammond, P. B. "Lead Poisoning: An Old Problem with a New Dimension." In F. R. Blood, ed., *Essays in Toxicology,* vol. 1. New York: 1964, pp. 115–155.

"Job Threats to Workers' Fertility Emerging as Civil Liberties Issue." *The New York Times,* January 15, 1979.

Kehoe, R. A. "Normal Metabolism of Lead." *Archives of Environmental Health* 8 (1964): 232–243.

"Lead Poisoning Perils Crew Razing El." *New York Times,* May 14, 1974.

"Lead Poisoning Takes a Big, Continuing Toll as Cures Prove Elusive." *Wall Street Journal,* May 27, 1982.

Lynam, Donald R., Piantanida, L., and Cole, J., eds. *Environmental Lead.* New York: 1981. Scientific papers from a 1978 symposium.

Marshall, Eliot. "Legal Threat Halts CDC Meeting on Lead." *Science* 223 (1984): 672.

Murozumi, M., Chow, Tsaihwa, and Patterson, C. "Chemical Concentrations of Pollutant Lead Aerosols, Terrestrial Dusts and Sea Salts in Greenland and Antarctic Snow Strata." *Geochemica et Cosmochimica Acta* 33 (1969): 1247–1294.

*National Research Council. Committee on Lead in the Human Environment. *Lead in the Human Environment.* Washington, D.C.: 1980.

Needleman, H. L. "The Lead We Breathe." *New York Times,* February 23, 1974.

* ———, ed. *Low Level Lead Exposure: The Clinical Implications of Current Research.* New York: 1980.

Nriagu, Jerome. "Saturnine Gout among Roman Aristocrats." *The New England Journal of Medicine* 308 (1983): 660–663.

Oehme, F. W., ed. *Toxicity of Heavy Metals in the Environment.* New York: 1978.

Patterson, C. C. "Contaminated and Natural Lead Environments of Man." *Archives of Environmental Health* 11 (1965): 344–360.

*Ramazzini, Bernardino. *Diseases of Workers.* New York: 1964. The great original classic work on occupational diseases. Should engage anyone interested in medicine, the environment, the workplace, and the history of science.

Reece, Robert. "Childhood Lead Poisoning: A Preventable Disaster." *American Family Physician* 9 (1974): 136–140.

Sayre, James, et al. "House and Hand Dust as a Potential Source of Childhood Lead Exposure." *American Journal of Diseases of Children* 127 (1974): 167–170.

Schroeder, Henry, and Tipton, Isabel. "The Human Body Burden of Lead." *Archives of Environmental Health* 17 (1968): 965–978.

Singhal, R. L., and Thomas, J. A., eds. *Lead Toxicity.* Baltimore: 1980.

Steinbock, R. Ted. "Lead Ingestion in Ancient Times." *Paleopathology Newsletter* No. 27 (1979): 9–11.

Tanquerel des Planches, L. *Traité des Maladies de Plomb ou Saturnines.* Paris: 1839.

Thomas, H. V., et al. "Blood Lead of Persons Living Near Freeways." *Archives of Environmental Health* 15 (1967): 695–702.

Trotter, Robert, et al. "Arcazon and *Greta:* Ethnomedical Solution to Epidemiological Mystery." *Medical Anthropology Quarterly* 14 (1983): 3, 18.

Vitruvius. *The Ten Books on Architecture.* New York: 1960. One of many Roman sources on the use of lead.

Waldron, H. A., and Stofen, D. *Sub-Clinical Lead Poisoning.* New York: 1976. A good work with a good bibliography.

Wessel, Morris, and Dominski, Anthony. "Our Children's Daily Lead." *American Scientist* 65 (1977): 294–299.

Chapter 8: The Upright, the Erotic

Unfortunately, much of the material central to this chapter is scattered in specialized journals and collections of papers. Still, there are some good works available to laymen, such as those by Harlow, Diamond and Karlen, Karlen, Eibl-Eibesfeldt, Singer, and Tinbergen. The book by Symons is a good recent summary of research for specialists, and the papers of Frank Beach are always valuable. Tiger's article is thoughtful and failed to receive the national attention it deserved. My thanks to Dr. Timothy Perper for his research material and his help.

Bateson, Patrick, ed. *Mate Choice*. New York: 1983. Good collection of recent essays, for specialists.
Beach, Frank A. "Sexual Attractivity, Proceptivity, and Receptivity in Female Mammals." *Hormones and Behavior* 7 (1976): 105–138. A major scientific paper.
———. "Human Sexuality and Evolution." In W. Montagna and W. A. Sadler, eds., *Reproductive Behavior*. New York: 1974.
*———, ed. *Human Sexuality in Four Perspectives*. Baltimore: 1977. Important for the advanced reader.
———, ed. *Sex and Behavior*. New York: 1965. Still an important collection of research papers, for specialists.
Buffum, John, et al. "Drugs and Sexual Function." In Harold Lief, ed., *Sexual Problems in Medical Practice*. Chicago: 1981, pp. 211–242.
Burton, F. D. "Sexual Climax in Female Macaca Mulatta." *Proceedings of the Third International Congress of Primatology, Zurich, 1970*. 3 (1970): 180–191.
Chevalier-Skolnikoff, S. "Male-Male, Female-Female, and Male-Female Sexual Behavior in the Stumptail Monkey, with Special Attention to the Female Orgasm." *Archives of Sexual Behavior* 3 (1974): 95–116.
*Diamond, Milton, and Karlen, Arno. *Sexual Decisions*. Boston: 1980. A text meant for undergraduates but also used in some medical and nursing schools. The authors think it is good. Extensive bibliography.
*Eibl-Eibesfeldt, Irenius. *Love and Hate*. New York: 1974. An excellent introduction for laymen to the evolutionary roots of human behavior.
Fisher, A. "Chemical and Electrical Stimulation of the Brain in the Male Rat." In R. A. Gorski and R. Whalen, eds., *Brain and Behavior*, vol. 3. Berkeley: 1966.
Fox, C. A., and Fox, B. "A Comparative Study of Coital Physiology, with Special Reference to the Sexual Climax." *Journal of Reproduction and Fertility* 24 (1971): 319–336.
Ford, Clellan, and Beach, Frank. *Patterns of Sexual Behavior*. New York: 1951. Dated and flawed, but still useful.
*Harlow, Harry. *Learning to Love*. New York: 1974. A readable summary for laymen of a great psychologist's studies. The bibliography directs one to the research papers on which the book is based.

Hutt, Corinne. *Males and Females*. Baltimore: 1972. Good introduction to the study of sex differences.

Jonas, David, and Jonas, Doris. *Sex and Status*. New York: 1975.

Karlen, Arno. *Sexuality and Homosexuality: A New View*. New York: 1971. Several chapters on the roots of courtship, sex differences, and the evolution of behavior. Extensive critical bibliography.

Kinsey, Alfred, et al. *Sexual Behavior in the Human Female*. Philadelphia: 1953. Still indispensable.

Lehrman, Daniel. "Interaction between Internal and External Environments in the Reproduction of the Ring Dove." In Beach, *Sex and Behavior* (above), pp. 355–380.

Lowry, Thomas, and Lowry, Thea. *The Clitoris*. St. Louis: 1976. A useful compendium of biological and cultural information.

Masters, William, and Johnson, Virginia. *Human Sexual Response*. Boston: 1966. Still indispensable.

———. "Human Sexual Inadequacy and Some Parameters of Therapy." In Milton Diamond, ed., *Perspectives in Reproductive and Sexual Behavior*. Bloomington: 1968, pp. 411–415.

Michael, Richard. "Neuroendrocrine Factors Regulating Primate Behaviour." In L. Martini and W. F. Ganong, eds., *Frontiers in Neuroendocrinology*. New York: 1971.

Michael, Richard, and Zumpe, Doris. "Potency in Male Rhesus Monkeys." *Science* 200 (1978): 451–453.

Morris, Desmond. *The Human Zoo*. New York: 1969. Despite questionable generalizations, this book and Morris's *The Naked Ape* made many people aware of ethology as a light on human behavior.

*Perper, Timothy. *The Eyes of Love: The Biosocial Basis of Human Courtship*. Philadelphia: in press. A fascinating new study in human ethology.

Scheflen, Albert. *How Behavior Means*. New York: 1974. Good nontechnical book on body language.

Singer, Irving. *The Goals of Human Sexuality*. New York: 1973.

Symons, Don. *The Evolution of Human Sexuality*. Oxford: 1979. A good review for specialists, with a useful section on orgasm in nonhuman females.

Teitelbaum, Michael, ed. *Sex Differences: Social and Biological Perspectives*. Garden City: 1976. Good collection of medical and anthropological views for the serious lay reader.

Tiger, Lionel. "The Emotional Effects of the Pill." *Viva* 1 (November 1973), p. 42 ff.

*Tinbergen, Niko. *The Herring Gull's World*. New York: 1967. A delight.

Udry, J. R., and Morris, N. M. "Distribution of Coitus in the Human Menstrual Cycle." *Nature* 220 (1968): 593–596.

*Wickler, Wolfgang. *The Sexual Code*. New York: 1973. Good book for laymen on the evolution of sex behavior.

Zumpe, Doris, and Michael, Richard. "Effects of Ejaculations by Males on the Sexual Invitations of Female Rhesus Monkeys (Macaca Mulatta)." *Behaviour* 60 (1977): 260–277.

———. "The Clutching Reaction and Orgasm in the Female Rhesus Monkey." *Journal of Endocrinology* 40 (1968): 117–123.

Epilogue: The Limping Ape

For interesting information on malaria and some bibliographical suggestions, see the books by McNeill, Cartwright, and Burnet and White, listed among references for Chapter 6; see also Brothwell and Sandison, whose book is listed among references for Chapter 5. Interesting material on growing up male or female is in many books listed for Chapter 7. Clemens is quoted by Kerr; Hsü by "The Iridium Connection"; Kauffman by Lewin (1); Martin by Lewin (2). Four important papers on the catastrophe theory appeared in the March 16, 1984, issue of *Science* (only one is listed below, by Alvarez et al.).

Alvarez, Walter, et al. "Iridium Anomaly Approximately Synchronous with Terminal Eocene Extinctions." *Science* 216 (1982): 886–888.

———. "Evidence for a Major Meteorite Impact on the Earth 34 Million Years Ago: Implications for Eocene Extinctions." *Science* 216 (1982): 885–886.

———. "The End of the Cretaceous: Sharp Boundary or Gradual Transition?" *Science* 223 (1984): 1183–1185.

Bidstrup, P. L. *Toxicity of Mercury and Its Compounds*. Amsterdam: 1964.

Bolk, Ludwig. *Das Problem der Menschwerdung*. Jena: 1926. Quoted in Jonas and Klein (below).

Bowlby, John. *Attachment and Loss*. New York: 1969. A classic.

———. *Maternal Care and Maternal Health*. New York: 1967.

Broad, William. "Sir Isaac Newton: Mad as a Hatter." *Science* 213 (1981): 1341–1344.

Brown, A. C., and Crounse, R. G., eds. *Hair, Trace Elements and Human Illness*. New York: 1980.

deMause, Lloyd, ed. *The History of Childhood*. New York: 1974. Scholarly essays from the *Journal of Psychohistory*. Psychoanalytic-historical attempt to relate child-rearing and social patterns throughout history.

Ganapathy, R. "Evidence for a Major Meteorite Impact on the Earth

34 Million Years Ago: Implications for Eocene Extinctions." *Science* 216 (1982): 885–888.

Glass, B. F., and Zwart, M. H. In F. M. Swain, ed., *Stratigraphic Micropaleontology of Atlantic Basin and Borderlands.* Amsterdam: 1977.

Hsü, K. J., et al. "Mass Mortality and Its Environmental and Evolutionary Consequences." *Science* 216 (1982): 249–256.

"The Iridium Connection." *Scientific American* 243 (August 1980): 86B, 90.

Jonas, David, and Klein, Doris. *Man-Child.* New York: 1970. Fascinating combination of scientific review and speculation. For laymen.

Kerr, Richard. "Extinctions: Iridium and Who Went Where." *Science* 215 (1982): 389.

———. "Periodic Impacts and Extinctions Reported." *Science* 223 (1984): 1277–1279.

Lewin, Roger. "Extinctions and the History of Life." *Science* 221 (1983): 935–937.

———. "What Killed the Giant Mammals?" *Science* 221 (1983): 1036–1037.

Luck, J. M., and Turekian, K. K. "Osmium-187/Osmium-186 in Manganese Nodules and the Cretaceous-Tertiary Boundary." *Science* 216 (1982): 613–615.

Massie, Robert. *Nicholas and Alexandra.* New York: 1967. This popular book on the late Romanovs is well written. The bibliography on hemophilia is no longer up to date, but the book gives laymen a good introduction to the impact of hereditary disease.

Peiper, Albrecht. *Cerebral Function in Infancy and Childhood.* New York: 1963.

"Physical and Mental Disabilities in Newborns Doubled in 25 Years." *The New York Times,* July 18, 1983.

Rampino, Michael, and Reynolds, Robert. "Analysis of the Cretaceous-Tertiary Boundary Clay: Methodology Questioned." *Science* 223 (1984): 190–191.

Russell, Dale. "The Mass Extinctions of the Late Mesozoic." *Scientific American* 246 (1982): 58–65.

Spargo, P. E., and Pounds, C. A. *Notes and Records of the Royal Society of London* 34 (1979): 11. On Newton and Mercury.

Westfall, Richard. *Never at Rest.* New York: 1981. Biography of Newton.

Index